VEGAN BODYBUILDING COOKBOOK 2021

Quick and Easy High-Protein Plant-Based Recipes

FOR VEGAN&VEGETARIAN BODYBUILDERS, ATHLETES, FITNESS AND SPORTS ENTHUSIAST

Balanced Plant-Based Sports Nutrition

Copyright © 2021

All rights reserved

No part of this publication may be reproduced or distributed in any form or by any means, electronic or mechanical, or stored in a database or retrieval system, without prior written permission from the publisher.

The authors are not licensed practitioners, physicians, or medical professionals and offer no medical diagnoses, treatments, suggestions, or counseling. The information presented herein has not been evaluated by the U.S. Food and Drug Administration, and it is not intended to diagnose, treat, curt, or prevent any disease. Full medical clearance from a licensed physician should be obtained before beginning or modifying any diet, exercise, or lifestyle program, and physicians should be informed of all nutritional changes.

The authors/owners claim no responsibility to any person or entity for any liability, loss, or damage caused or alleged to be caused directly or indirectly as a result of the use, application, or interpretation of the information presented herein.

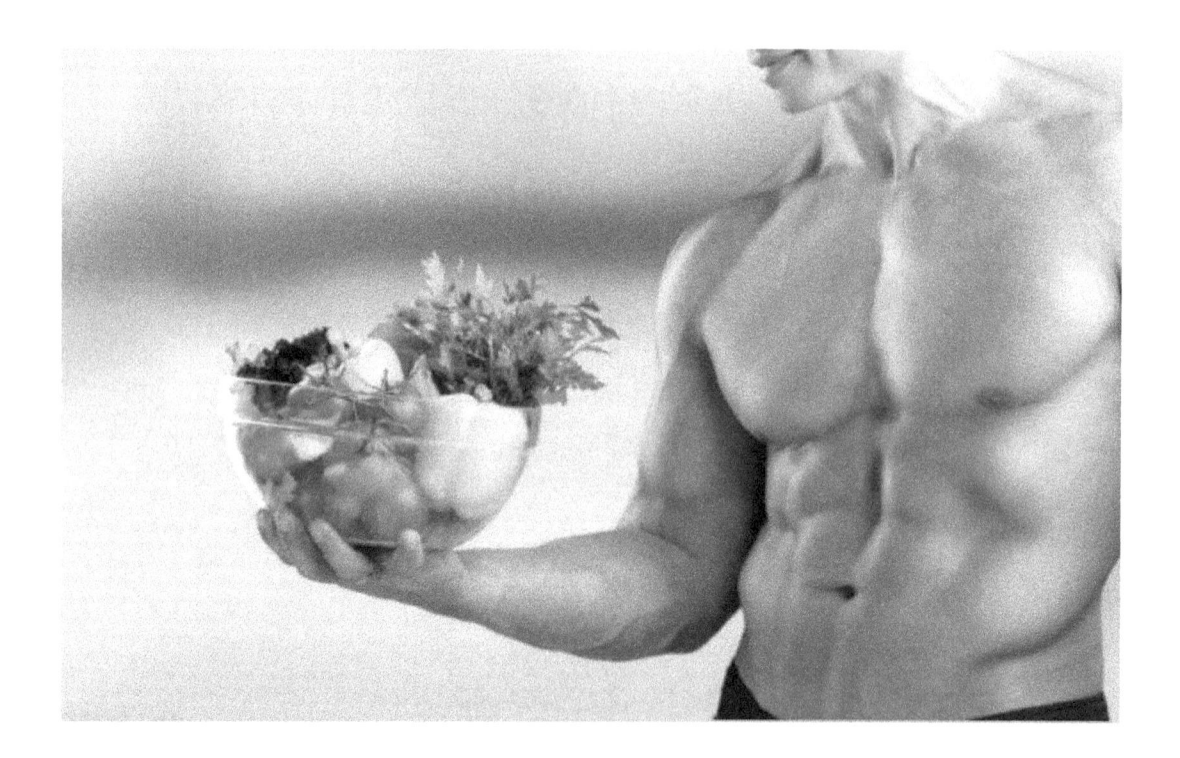

Introduction

What Can a Vegetarian Eat?

    Foods to Avoid

    "Blacklist" foods for Vegetarian

Best Protein Sources for Vegetarian Athletes

    TOP vegetarian protein sources

    Legumes

    Nuts

    Seeds

The Principle of Mutual Complementation of Proteins

How Much Protein do Athletes and Bodybuilders Need?

Proteins, Fats, and Carbohydrates for Vegetarian Athletes VEGAN COOKBOOK for BODYBUILDERS and ATHLETES High Energy Breakfasts

    Blueberry Banana Chia Oatmeal

    Banana StrawberrY Oats

    Avocado Sweet Potato Toast

    Banana Quinoa Oatmeal

    Spinach Tofu Scramble

    Hemp Seeds oatmeal

    Chocolate Breakfast Quinoa

    Banana Cauliflower Porridge

    Chai Flavoured Quinoa

Protein Salad

- Peanut Noodle Salad
- Broccoli Edamame Salad
- Black Bean Lentil Salad
- Tomato Green Lentil Salad
- Arugula Green Beans Salad
- Sorghum Kale Pesto Salad
- Red Cabbage Salad
- Quinoa Chickpeas Avocado Salad
- Butternut Squash Spinach Salad
- White Bean & Avocado Salad
- Spring Watermelon Radish Salad

Savory Protein Snacks

- Choc Chickpea Cookies
- Cherry Vanilla Protein Bars
- Kale Paprika Chips
- Vanilla Almonds Hemp Protein Bars
- Spicy Squash Seeds

Soups

- Basic Recipe for Vegetable Broth
- Creamy White Bean Soup
- Spicy Sun-dried Tomato Soup
- Creamy Black Bean Soup

Farro Lentil Soup

Greek Lentil Soup

Pumpkin & White Bean Soup

Creamy Broccoli Soup with Chickpeas

Carrot & Red Lentil Soup

Lunch & Dinner

Red Cabbage Tacos

Spaghetti Squash with Tempeh

Vegan Chili Carne

Vegan Tofu Spinach Lasagne

Sesame Tofu with Soba Noodles

Mexican Green Lentis Soup

Lemon Fettucine Alfredo

Quinoa Bowls with Spiralized

Zucchini Sweet & Sour Tempeh

Desserts for a Good Mood

Vanilla Chia Quinoa Pudding

Chocolate Chia Pudding

Banana Peanut Butter Oatmeal

Pumpkin Pie Pudding

Banana Cacao Ice Cream

High-Protein Smoothie

Berry Recovery Protein Smoothie

[Green High Protein Smoothie](#)

[Banana Mango Smoothie](#)

[Banana Avocado and Hempseed Smoothie](#)

[Banana Strawberry Chia Smoothie](#)

INTRODUCTION

Do you often hear comments such as:

- Oh, are you a vegan athlete? Where do you get protein from?

- Bodybuilder vegan? C'mon ... It can't be!

- Building muscle without meat? It's impossible!

If you're a vegan, you've probably heard these a million times.

So is it possible to follow a vegetarian way of life and do sports, fitness or bodybuilding at the same time? Are vegetarianism and sports compatible?

We present you a book for vegetarian athletes, bodybuilders, fitness, and sports enthusiast, written by a nutritionist, vegetarian, and trainer on healthy eating.

Vegan athletes, bodybuilders, fitness or sports enthusiast have special dietary needs. Vegans working out with the to rebuild their body, have to be extra vigilant of their protein intake and expenditure.

A vegetarian diet gives the body no less energy than a meat diet. You just need to keep track of the variety of foods consumed daily to ensure the right set of nutrients.

So, this book will help you in this matter.

In this VEGAN COOKBOOK, the author has collated the best high-protein plant-based recipes optimized for athletes, bodybuilders, any fitness or sports enthusiast, and men and women for balanced sports nutrition.

These easy-to-cook vegan recipes are suitable for anyone new to the vegan diet or cooking and will allow you to reduce your time in the kitchen in order to pay more attention to your workouts:

- High protein breakfasts for energy

- Protein salads with healthy nutrients

- First courses for proper nutrition

- Delicious staple foods for energy recovery
- Savory snacks and protein smoothies
- Plant-based protein desserts for a good

mood All recipes include full macro profiles.

In addition, in the first chapters of this book, we recall the basic and important aspects of a vegetarian diet for vegetarian athletes, bodybuilders, sports and fitness enthusiasts.

Gain muscle mass by eating properly and recharge your batteries for your sporting achievements!

Starting a vegetarian diet is a great idea, but you have to know where and how to start this process.

There is so much different and conflicting information about vegetarianism and sports compatible - how do you find the right answers to all your questions?

We provided all the necessary facts about the vegetarian plant-based diet in general and, in particular, about the rules for protein intake for vegan athletes, bodybuilders, fitness or sports enthusiasts in our book. In this book, we will talk about the basics of a plant-based diet and everything you need to know when starting out. Also, in this book, we share with you simple and easy steps on how to start a vegetarian plant-based diet without harm to your health. And these simple steps will help you to achieve your goal!

So, from this book you will learn:
- What is vegetarianism itself all about? What is veganism?
- How can you devote yourself to that? What would it cost you?
- What is the nicest way to turn down meat?
- Foods for a vegan diet - what you can and cannot eat?
- Best high protein sources on a vegan diet
- Vitamins and supplements for athletes and bodybuilders on a vegan diet
- How to start a vegan diet?
- The basics of vegan diets (calories, proteins, carbohydrates, fats, vitamins and minerals) for athletes and bodybuilders
- How much protein you need for your workouts?
- How to gain weight on a vegan diet?
- How can you still build muscle?

Learn how to easily switch from an animal diet to healthier plant-based food without sacrificing delicious foods.

In the following chapters, we recall the main and important aspects of a vegetarian diet for vegetarian athletes, bodybuilders, sports and fitness enthusiasts.

WHAT CAN A VEGETARIAN EAT?

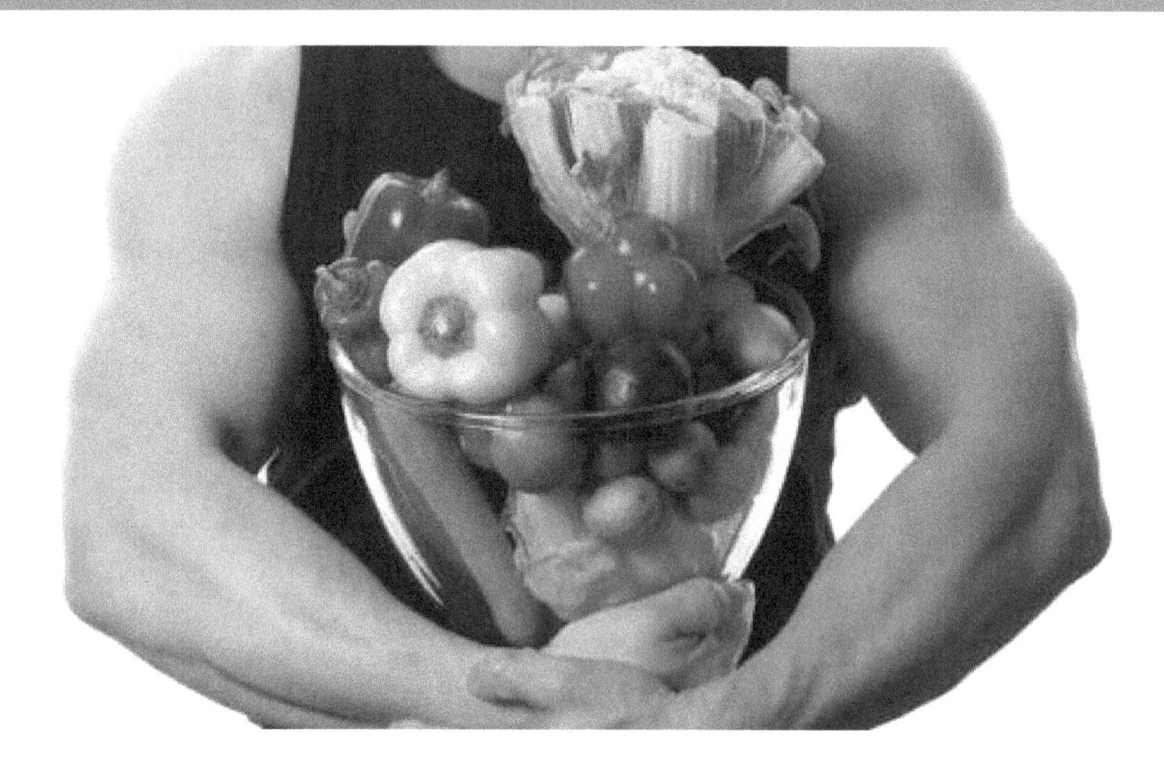

When you finally decide to follow a vegetarian plant-based diet, below is a list of foods you can consume:

- Vegetables: Carrots, kale, pepper, tomatoes, spinach, asparagus, broccoli, cauliflower, etc.
- Whole Grains: Rolled oats, quinoa, brown rice, brown rice pasta, farro, etc.
- Fruits: Pears, bananas, apples, berries, peaches, mangoes, pineapples etc.
- Legumes: Chickpeas, peas, black beans, peanuts,
- lentils, etc. Starchy Vegetables: Sweet potatoes, butternut squash, potatoes, etc.
- Nuts, Seeds and Nut Butters: Tahini, almonds, sunflower seeds, macadamia nuts, natural peanut butter, pumpkin seeds, etc.

- Healthy Fats: Olive oil, unsweetened coconut, avocados, coconut oil, etc.
- Condiments: Mustard, soy sauce, lemon juice, salsa, nutritional yeast, vinegar, etc.
- Plant-based Protein: Tempeh, Tofu, plant-based protein sources, etc.
- Unsweetened Plant-based Milks: Almond milk, cashew milk, coconut milk, etc.
- Spices, Seasonings, and Herbs: Rosemary, turmeric, black pepper, basil, curry, salt, etc.
- Beverages: Sparkling water, tea, coffee, etc.

FOODS TO AVOID

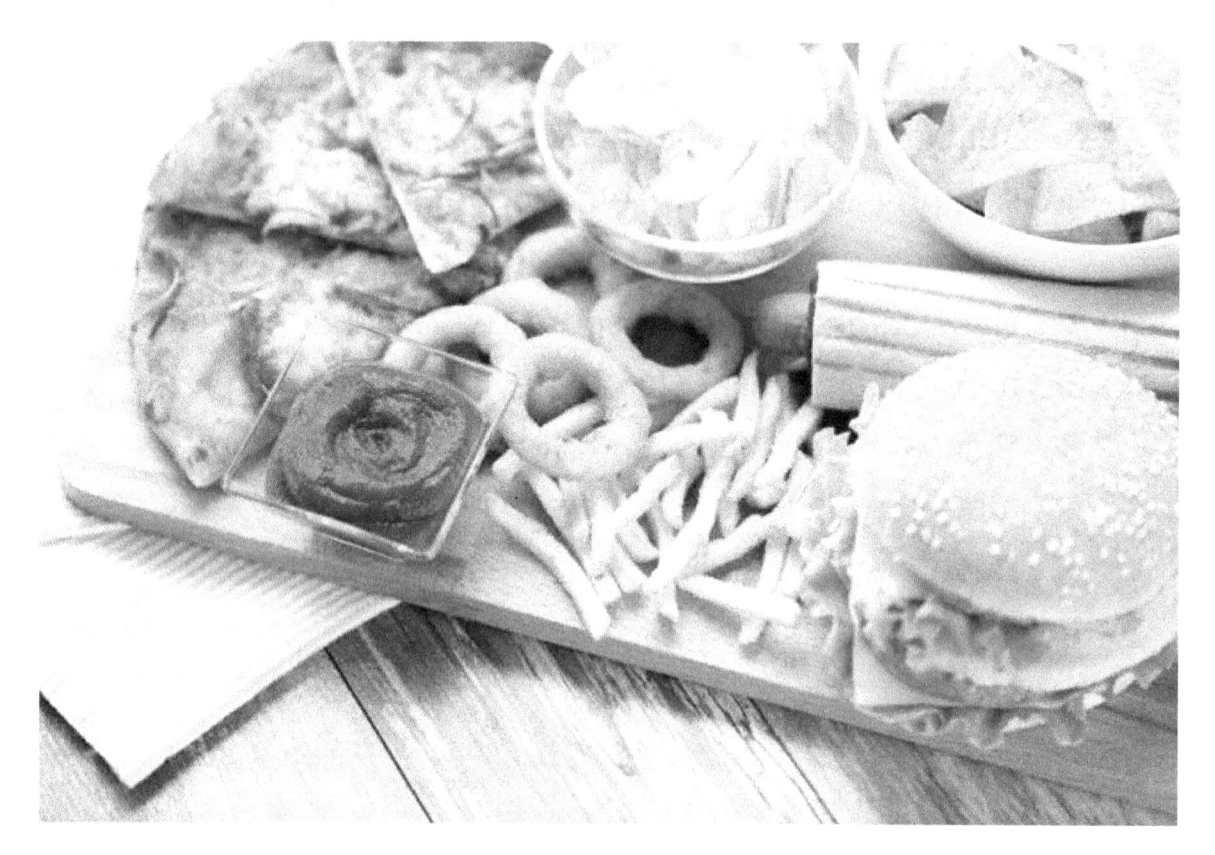

- Fast Food: Hotdogs, french fries, cheeseburgers, chicken nuggets, etc.
- Processed Animal Foods: Lunch meats, beef jerky, bacon, sausage, etc.
- Refined Grains: Bagels, white pasta, white rice, white bread, etc.
- Added Sugars and Sweets: Soda, sugary cereals, pastries, candy, cookies, table sugar, sweet tea, etc.
- Convenience and Packed Foods: Cereal bars, chips, frozen dinners, crackers, etc.

"BLACKLIST" FOODS FOR VEGETARIAN

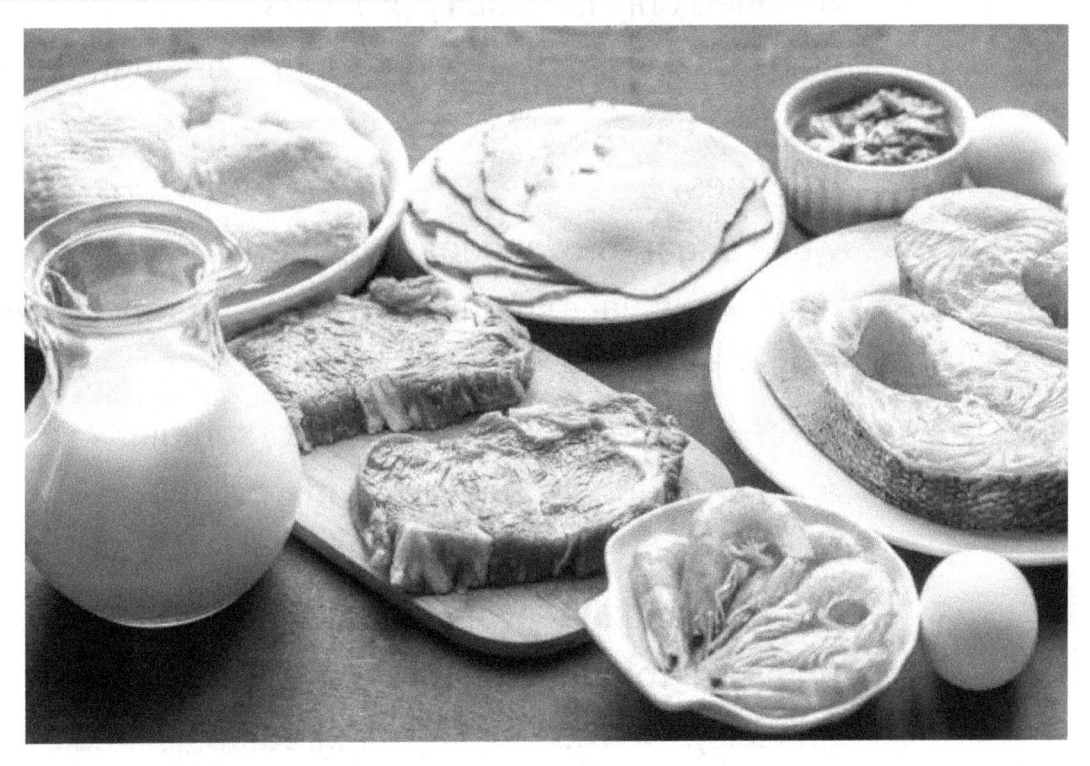

Many foods purchased in the store contain ingredients that either contain substances of animal origin, or, in one way or another, are associated with the exploitation of animals. In short, there are many foods that seem vegan, but vegans should avoid them.

Besides the commonly understood vegan no-nos, foods to say goodbye to forever include:

- all meat, poultry, and animal flesh;
- seafood;
- dairy products ;
- bee produced products like honey, beeswax, royal jelly, and pollen;
- food additives: some of them of animal origin, for example, E120, E322, E422, E 471, E542, E631, E901, and E904;

- dairy ingredients: whey, casein, and lactose are obtained only from dairy products;
chips (may contain chicken fat or dairy ingredients
- such as casein, whey or animal-derived enzymes);
- white sugar, brown sugar, powdered sugar (it is better to replace them with maple syrup or agave nectar as a sweetener);
- some varieties of dark chocolate (contain animal products - whey, milk fat, milk powder, refined oil or skimmed milk powder);
- red products that owe their color to red pigments obtained from the bodies of cochineal females (insects). On the label, this ingredient is labeled cochineal, carmine acid, or carmine;
- margarine (may contain gelatin, casein (milk protein) and whey);
- pasta (some types of pasta, especially fresh ones, contain eggs);
- non-dairy cream (many varieties of such cream contain milk protein casein);
- Worcestershire sauce (spicy soy sauce with vinegar and spices): many varieties contain anchovies;
- gelatin (a product of the processing of connective tissue of animals);
- pepsin (the enzyme is present in the gastric juice of mammals, birds, reptiles and most fish);

- Vitamin D3 (most vitamin D3 is derived from fish oil or lanolin, which is present in sheep's wool);

- Omega-3 fatty acids (the source of most omega-3s is fish).

BEST PROTEIN SOURCES FOR VEGETARIAN ATHLETES

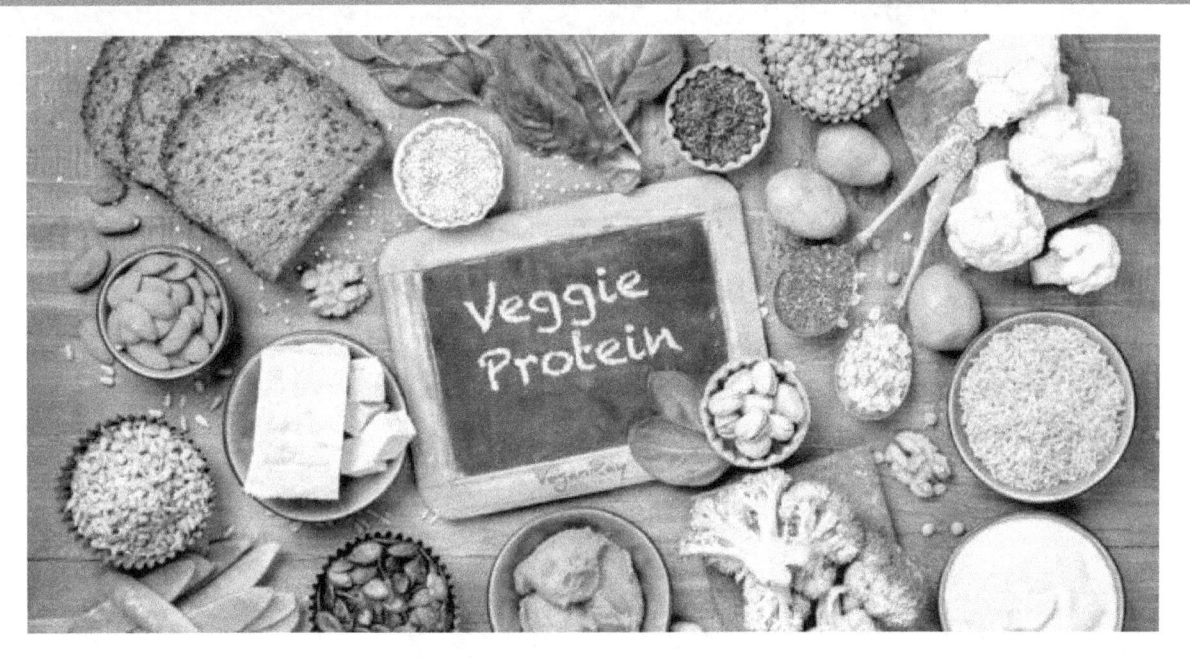

Vegan athletes and bodybuilders have special dietary needs. Vegans working out with the to rebuild their body, have to be extra vigilant of their protein intake.

The amount of protein that you need to eat depends on your exact workout routine, the type of your body, how long you have not eaten meat, and other factors.

When you systematically exercise, your need for protein increases. To become stronger so that muscles can recover effectively, it is necessary to provide them with a sufficient amount of building material - protein.

We all know that nature is an excellent source of protein.

So, we provide all the necessary facts about the best sources of protein for a vegan diet.

TOP VEGETARIAN PROTEIN SOURCES

PER 100G (3.5 OZ) IN WEIGHT

Food	Protein (g)
Potato	2.50
Brown Rice	2.58
Spinach	2.90
Quinoa	4.40
Kidney Beans	4.83
Pinto Beans	4.86
Green Peas	5.36
Macadamia Nuts	7.79
Lima Beans	7.80
Wheat Bread	8.80
Garbanzo Beans	8.90
Lentils	9.02
Pecans	9.50
Soybeans	13.10
Walnuts	15.03
Hazelnuts	15.03
Cashew Nuts	15.31
Chia Seeds	15.60
Oats	16.89
Tofu	17.19
Flaxseed	19.50
Pistachio Nuts	21.35
Almonds	22.09
Hemp Seed	23.00
Peanut Butter	25.09
Pumpkin Seeds	32.97

SO WHAT ARE HIGH PROTEIN PLANTS?

LEGUMES

Beans, pulses, lentils, chickpeas are legumes. So are peas, beans, peanuts and anything that grows in a pod. Legumes are high in protein but not high in fat, so they are generally consumed as a healthy choice for meeting protein requirements as they can be consumed in large quantities without adding too many calories.

black lentils
12 grams per
1/2 cup

split peas
8 grams per
1/2 cup

green lentils
9 grams per
1/2 cup

chickpeas
~8 grams per
1/2 cup

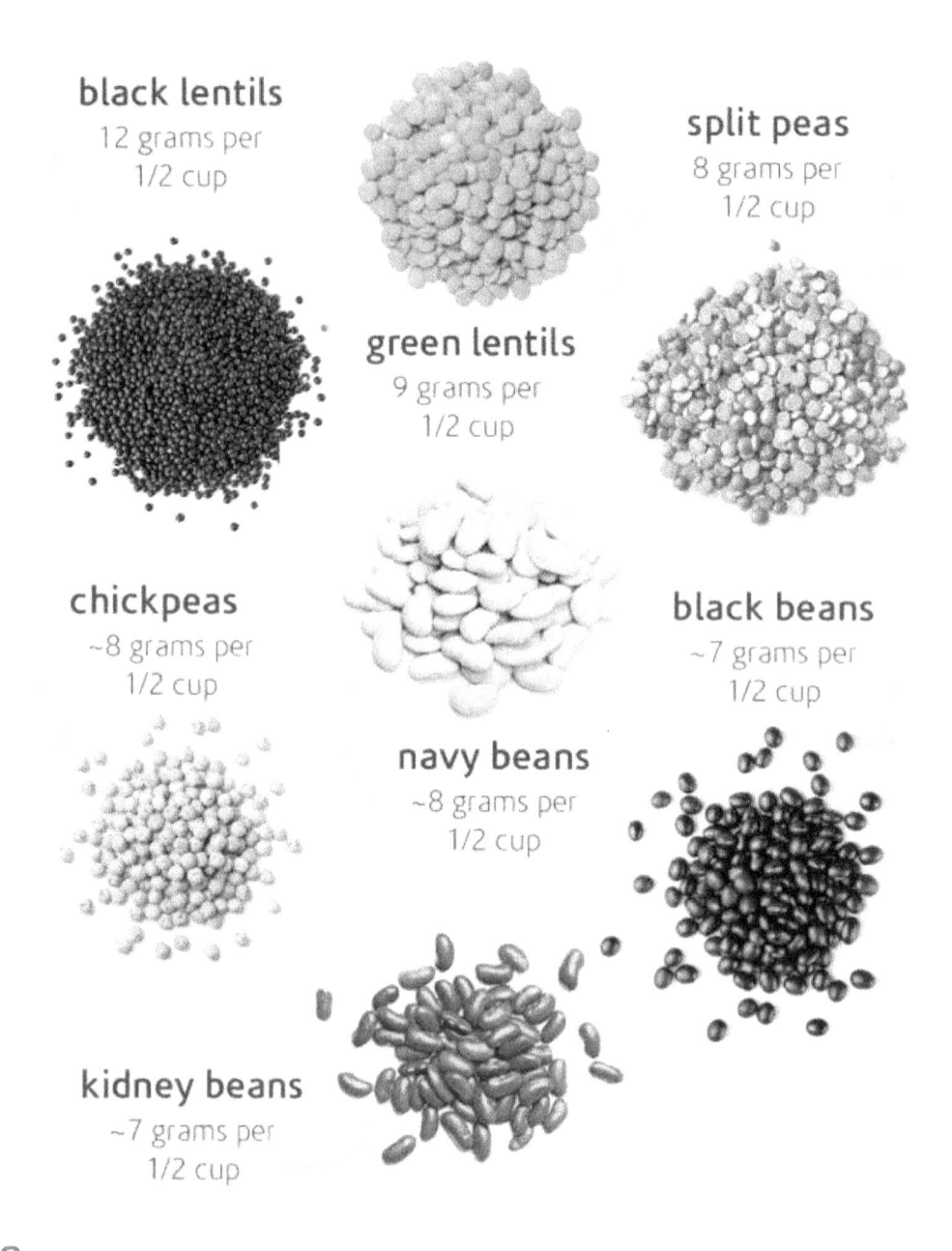

black beans
~7 grams per
1/2 cup

navy beans
~8 grams per
1/2 cup

kidney beans
~7 grams per
1/2 cup

BEANS

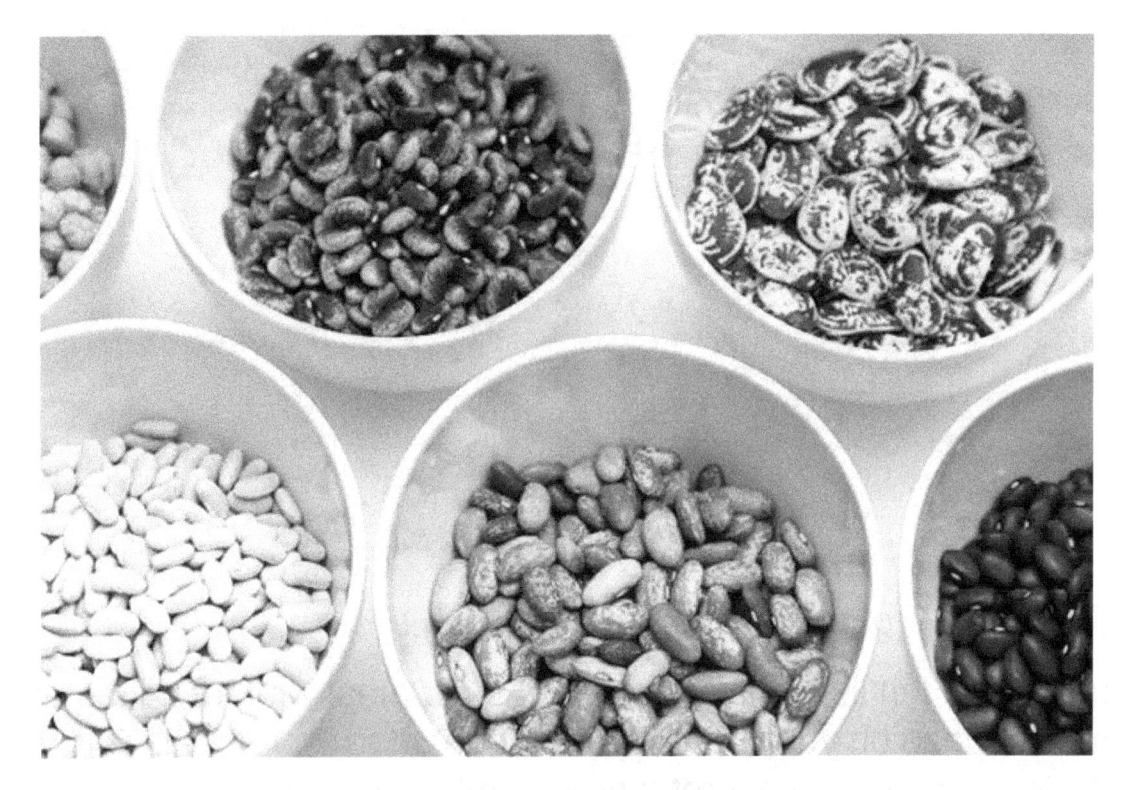

Beans are a popular vegan main source of protein, with the added benefit of slow digesting carbohydrates.

In the same category of high protein yield and low GI carbs you would also find pulses and lentils.

PULSES

While not exactly lentils, pulses are different in their botanical classification and not in their protein content.

Pea flour and pea protein is very popular as a protein shake additive for athletes and bodybuilders, and anyone generally needing to increase their protein intake in an easily digestible form.

LENTILS

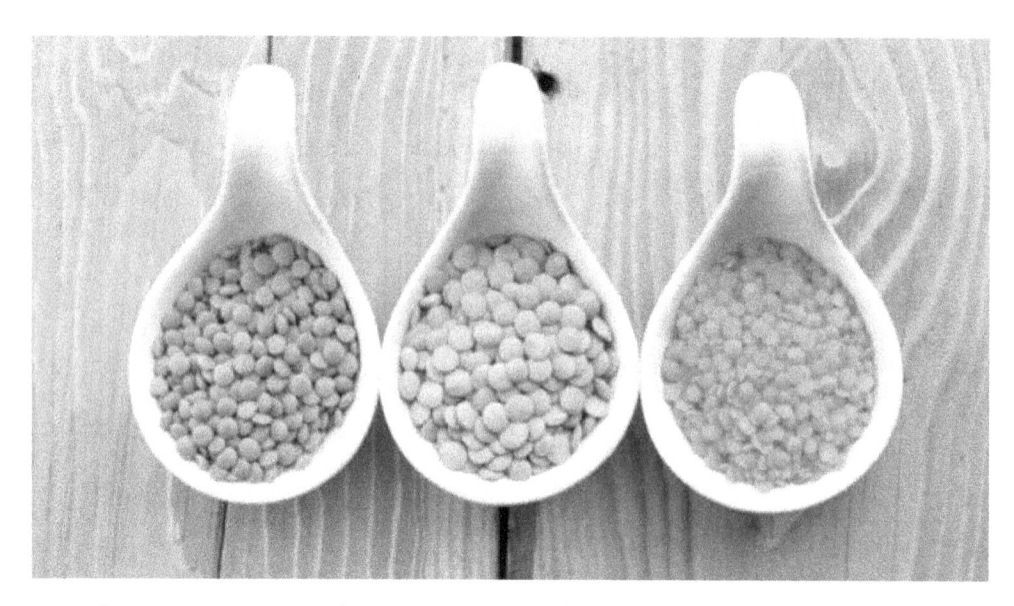

Lentils can be a great main course for lunch.

Legumes and lentils can add protein to your meal without taking up too much space on your plate if you add them to your meal. This is a good way to increase your total protein intake per meal.

CHICKPEAS

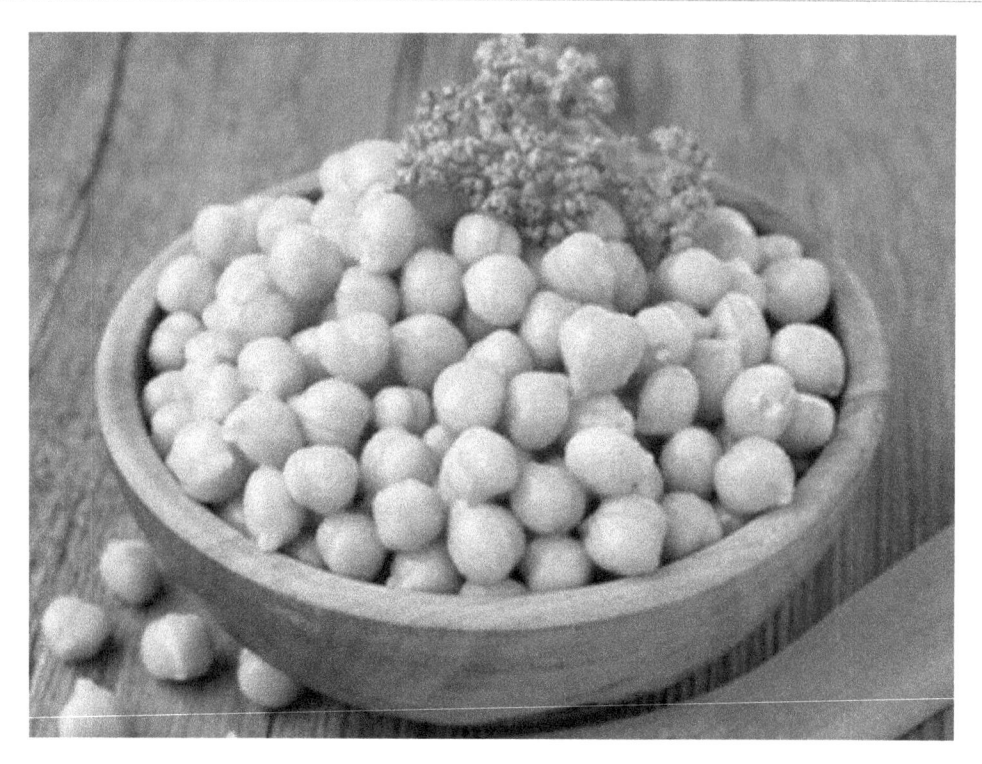

Chickpeas are high in protein, when cooked they contain around 14.5g protein per cup. Chickpeas can be eaten at any temperature and texture, and are highly versatile. Many traditional recipes that have been made for hundreds of years use these.

Hummus made from chickpeas is a great spread, dip or protein-rich puree. It's made from pureed chickpeas and provides B vitamins and protein in the diet. Use it as a butter to add protein to your plate.

NUTS

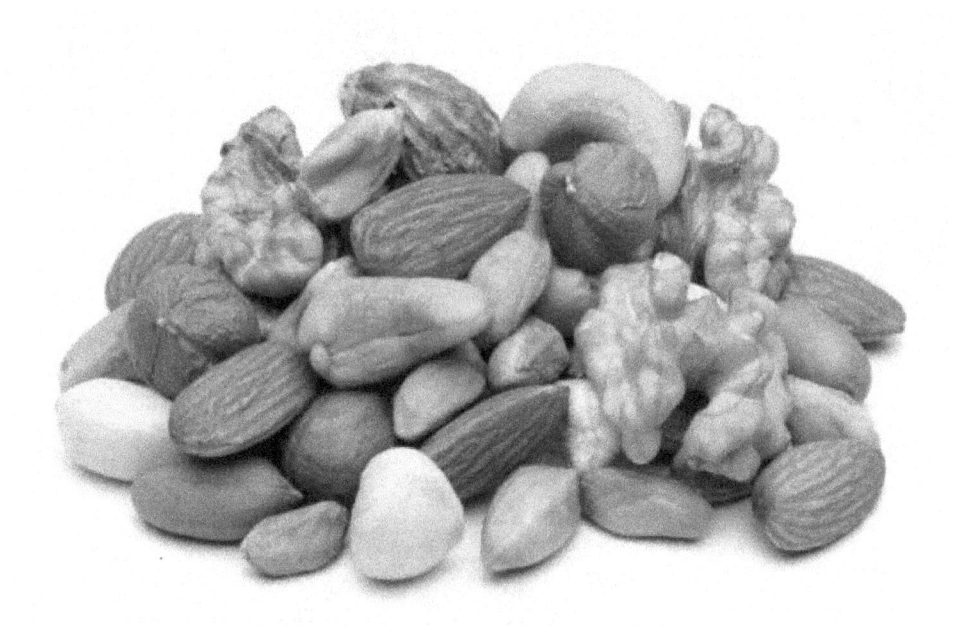

Examples of nuts are walnuts, cashews, almonds, Brazil nuts, peanuts, hazelnut, pistachios.

Peanuts are protein-rich, stuffed full of healthy fats, and can be beneficial to your cardiac health. Made into butter, peanuts are rich in protein, with 8 g per tablespoon, and versatile. Use it as a sandwich spread, added to smoothies, sauces and desserts.

Almonds contain a large amount of vitamin E, which is necessary for the health of nails, skin, and eyes. Walnuts are very good for brain health because of their protein profile.

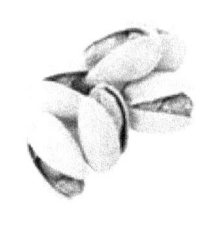

Pistachio (25g)
6g protein

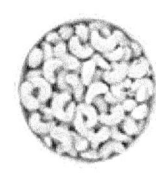

Cashew Nuts (25g)
4.5g protein

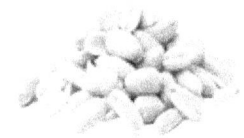

Peanuts (30g)
9g protein

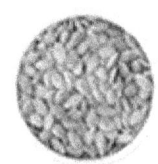

Pumpkin Seeds (25g)
7.5g protein

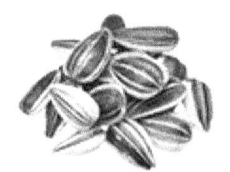

Sunflower Seeds (25g)
5g protein

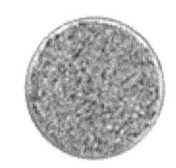

Flaxseed (30g)
6.6g protein

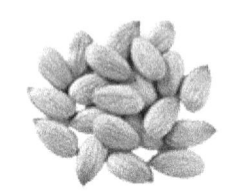

Almonds (25g)
5g protein

Chia Seeds (25g)
4g protein

SEEDS

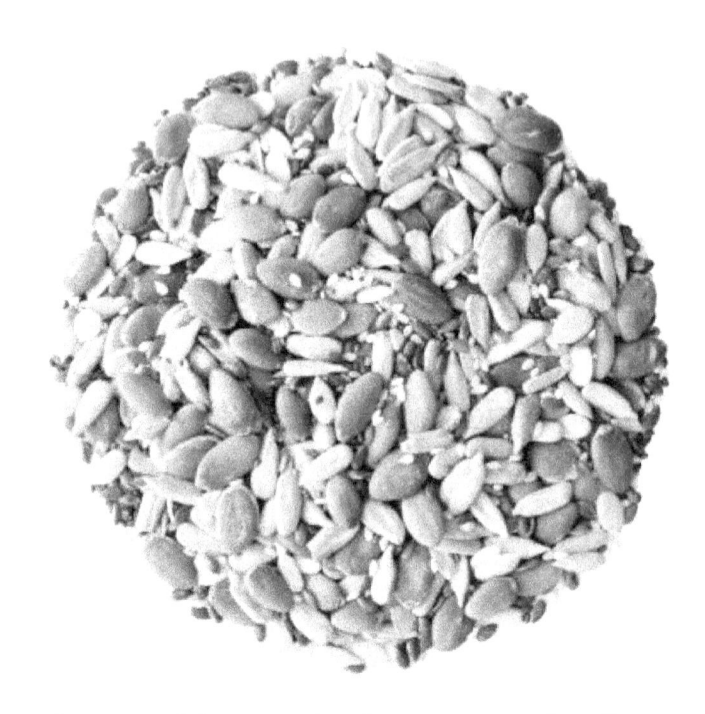

Examples of seeds are chia seeds, hemp seeds, flax seeds, sunflower and pumpkin seeds, peanuts seeds.

Seeds like quinoa are a complete protein. Other grains like millet, teff, amaranth, and sorghum also pack quite a large percentage of protein in a little package. They also make satisfying dense main ingredients to add to the main meal plate.

Flax seeds are high in Omegas and are a natural plant-derived and guilt-free way of getting your omega 3s and 6s.

Chia seeds are also high in protein and contain significant amounts of fiber. The tiny 'superfood' also has trace minerals Calcium, Manganese, Magnesium, and Phosphorous.

Hemp seeds are also a great protein source for people who get their protein from plants. Rich in fiber, protein and a range of fatty acids they also contain calcium, is a good source of plant-based iron, and magnesium.

QUINOA

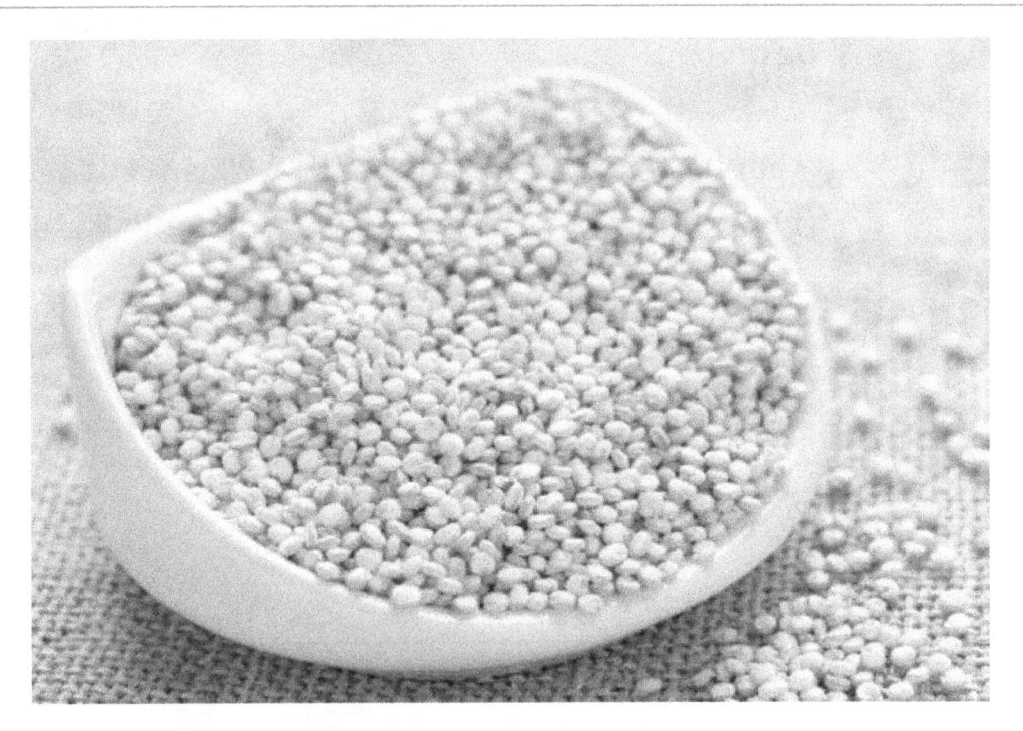

Quinoa is a seed (not a grain) with high fiber and surprisingly high protein content. Cooked quinoa contains 5 g of fiber and 8 g of protein per cup. The amino acids present in the seed form a complete protein, making it a unique plant food that is also rich in other nutrients, including magnesium, iron, and manganese.

This is a very versatile and super-nutritious food. Versatile because you can prepare it as a salad, main or breakfast. It can be sprouted or cooked to varying textures - firm, or softer for breakfasts and dessert dishes.

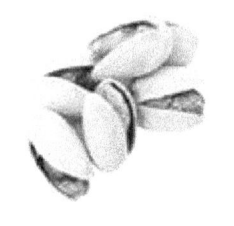

Pistachio (25g)
6g protein

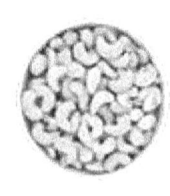

Cashew Nuts (25g)
4.5g protein

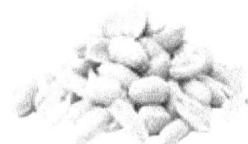

Peanuts (30g)
9g protein

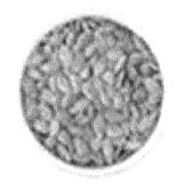

Pumpkin Seeds (25g)
7.5g protein

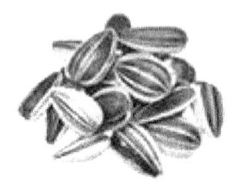

Sunflower Seeds (25g)
5g protein

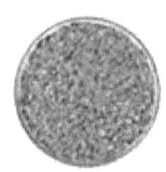

Flaxseed (30g)
6.6g protein

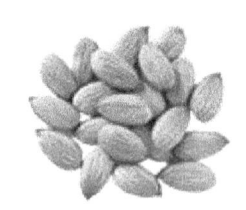

Almonds (25g)
5g protein

Chia Seeds (25g)
4g protein

THE PRINCIPLE OF MUTUAL COMPLEMENTATION OF PROTEINS

The secret of vegans is the principle of complementarity (mutual complement) of vegetable proteins. This principle implies the intake of two or three different types of plant foods, each of which partially contains different essential amino acids. Amino acids that are not present in one source of vegetable protein can be obtained from another. As a result of a combination of various sources of vegetable protein, we get the so-called complementary protein.

For example, breakfast consisting of lentil soup and wholemeal bread contains complementary amino acids that provide for the formation of a complete protein. Other examples are rice and beans, corn porridge or cornbread, and stewed beans.

A dish prepared from correctly selected plant components provides a complete set of complete proteins for muscle growth.

It is worth emphasizing that there is no need for each meal to carefully combine plant sources of protein to achieve the complementarity of essential amino acids. The main goal is to consume a sufficient number of different sources of vegetable protein, which will complement each other, distributing their consumption throughout the day.

For example, if you eat low-methionine beans for breakfast, and then snack on almonds rich in this amino acid, you get the right amount of methionine.

Pay particular attention to sesame seeds, sunflowers seeds, and pumpkin seeds, as well as tofu. These foods are especially rich in Branched Chain Amino Acids (BCAAs), which help reduce muscle damage after training and are actively involved in protein synthesis.

Complete Protein Guide for Vegetarians

Legumes

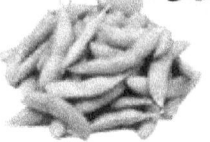

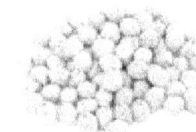

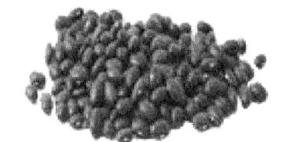

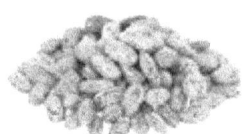

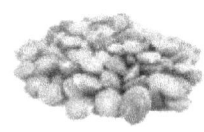

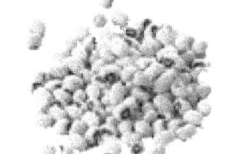

- Edamame
- Chickpeas
- Black Beans
- Pinto Beans
- Split Peas
- Black Eyed Peas
- Lentils
- Lima Beans

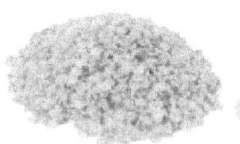

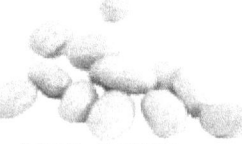

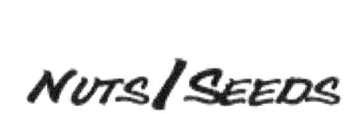

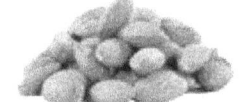

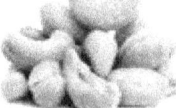

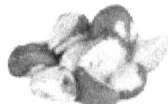

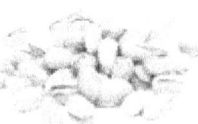

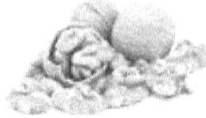

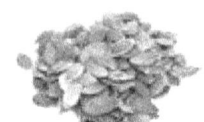

+

Nuts/Seeds

- Almonds
- Cashews
- Brazil Nuts
- Pistachios
- Walnuts
- Pumpkin Seeds
- Sesame Seeds
- Flaxseed

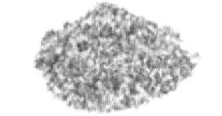

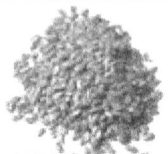

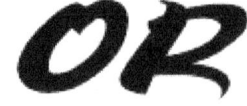

OR

Grains

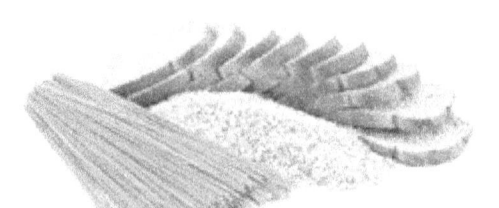

Whole wheat pita, bread, bun, rice or pasta

HOW MUCH PROTEIN DO ATHLETES AND

BODYBUILDERS NEED?

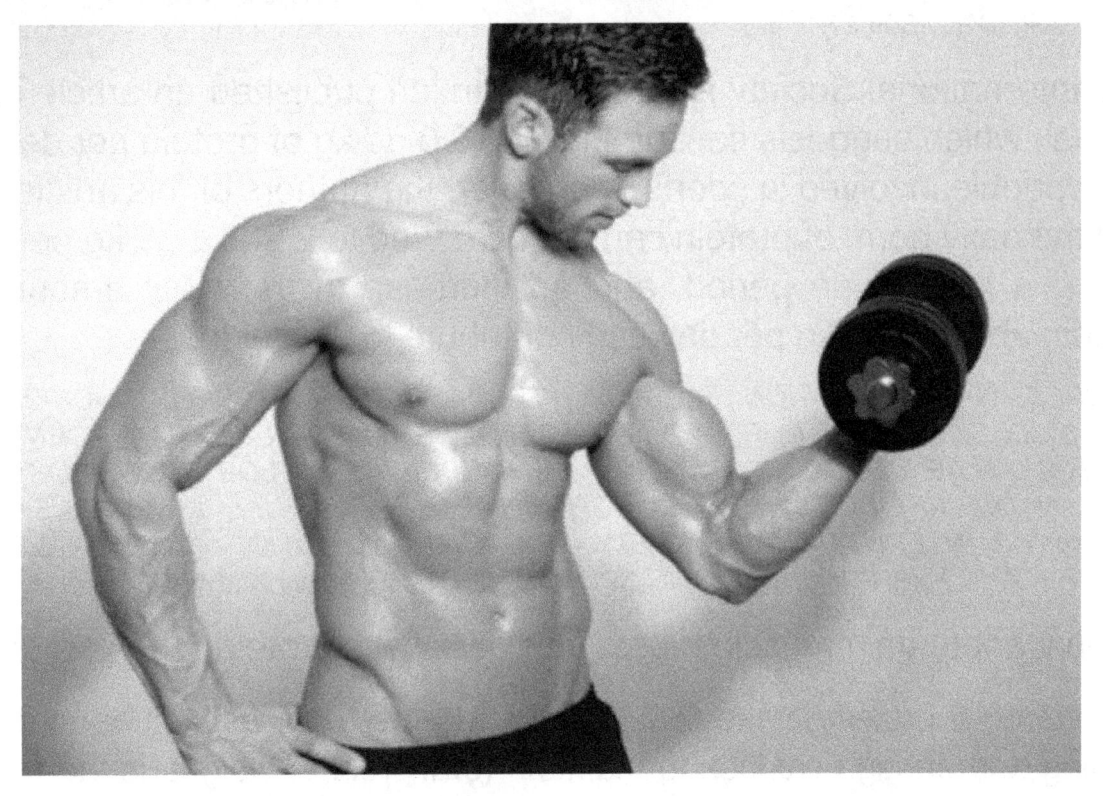

When you systematically exercise, your need for protein increases. To become stronger so that muscles can recover effectively, it is necessary to provide them with a sufficient amount of building material - protein.

The answer to this question is given by the authors of a study published in the International Journal of Sports Medicine:

- if you are engaged in power sports, then 1.4–1.8 g / kg per day;

- if you are fond of running or other endurance sports, then 1.2–1.4 g / kg per day.

(SOURCE OF INFORMATION: LEMON PW. DO ATHLETES NEED MORE DIETARY PROTEIN AND AMINO ACIDS? INT J SPORT NUTR. 1995 JUN;5 SUPPL:S39-61.)

The recommendations are consistent with the values published in the practice guide of the American College of Sports Medicine.

(SOURCE OF INFORMATION: RODRIGUEZ NR, DIMARCO NM, LANGLEY S; AMERICAN DIETETIC ASSOCIATION; DIETITIANS OF CANADA; AMERICAN COLLEGE OF SPORTS MEDICINE: NUTRITION AND ATHLETIC PERFORMANCE. POSITION OF THE AMERICAN

DIETETIC ASSOCIATION, DIETITIANS OF CANADA, AND THE AMERICAN COLLEGE OF SPORTS MEDICINE: NUTRITION AND ATHLETIC PERFORMANCE. J AM DIET ASSOC. 2009 MAR;109(3):509-27.).

The International Society for Sports Nutrition published an article in its journal, which suggests consuming 1.4–2.0 g / kg of protein per day for most people involved in sports. Moreover, the authors of this article say that the daily norm of protein can be increased to 2.3–3.1 g / kg per day during a low-calorie period, and an increase in the daily amount of protein above 3 g / kg per day can contribute to weight loss!

(SOURCE OF INFORMATION: JÄGER R, KERKSICK CM, CAMPBELL BI, CRIBB PJ, WELLS SD, SKWIAT TM, PURPURA M, ZIEGENFUSS TN, FERRANDO AA, ARENT SM, SMITH-RYAN AE, STOUT JR, ARCIERO PJ, ORMSBEE MJ, TAYLOR LW, WILBORN CD, KALMAN DS, KREIDER RB, WILLOUGHBY DS, HOFFMAN JR, KRZYKOWSKI JL, ANTONIO J. INTERNATIONAL SOCIETY OF SPORTS NUTRITION POSITION STAND: PROTEIN AND EXERCISE. J INT SOC SPORTS NUTR. 2017 JUN 20;14:20.)

If you want to gain muscle mass, you need less protein than you think.

In general, a protein intake of 0.8–1.2 g / kg per day, as well as strength training and enough calories to maintain (or increase) weight, is the recipe for building muscle that you need. Why do we need such a seemingly not very large amount of protein per day for weight gain? The fact is that most visitors to gyms do not receive any additional benefits when consuming more than 1.7 g / kg of protein per day. Moreover, this amount can even decrease with the accumulation of experience, since with regular weight lifting, the body reacts better and there is muscle damage.

A study published in the Journal of Applied Physiology, in which 12 novice bodybuilders took part, evaluated the 4-week effect of consuming 2.6 or 1.35 g / kg of protein per day. The researchers did not find any differences in strength or muscle growth between the two groups.

(SOURCE OF INFORMATION: LEMON PW, TARNOPOLSKY MA, MACDOUGALL JD, ATKINSON SA. PROTEIN REQUIREMENTS AND MUSCLE MASS/STRENGTH CHANGES DURING INTENSIVE TRAINING IN NOVICE BODYBUILDERS. J APPL PHYSIOL (1985). 1992 AUG;73(2):767-75.)

However, it should be remembered that such studies evaluate the short-term effect, while the long-term impact is studied much less frequently.

Here's the rule for you: consume enough protein, but remember that "the more you eat, the better" does not work: you are more likely to consume extra unnecessary calories. Remember the nutritional balance.

The recommendations for the optimal amount of daily protein are different and may depend on various factors. To maintain sufficient flexibility in your diet, try to consume from 0.8 to 1.8 g / kg of protein per day, based on your goals: weight gain, reduction in fat percentage, maintaining lean body mass. In addition, it is crucial to consider your training load, training conditions, eating habits, food availability and several other factors. Perhaps you need extra protein to feel full, or, conversely, you need to reduce protein intake and calories in general.

PROTEINS, FATS, AND CARBOHYDRATES FOR VEGETARIAN ATHLETES

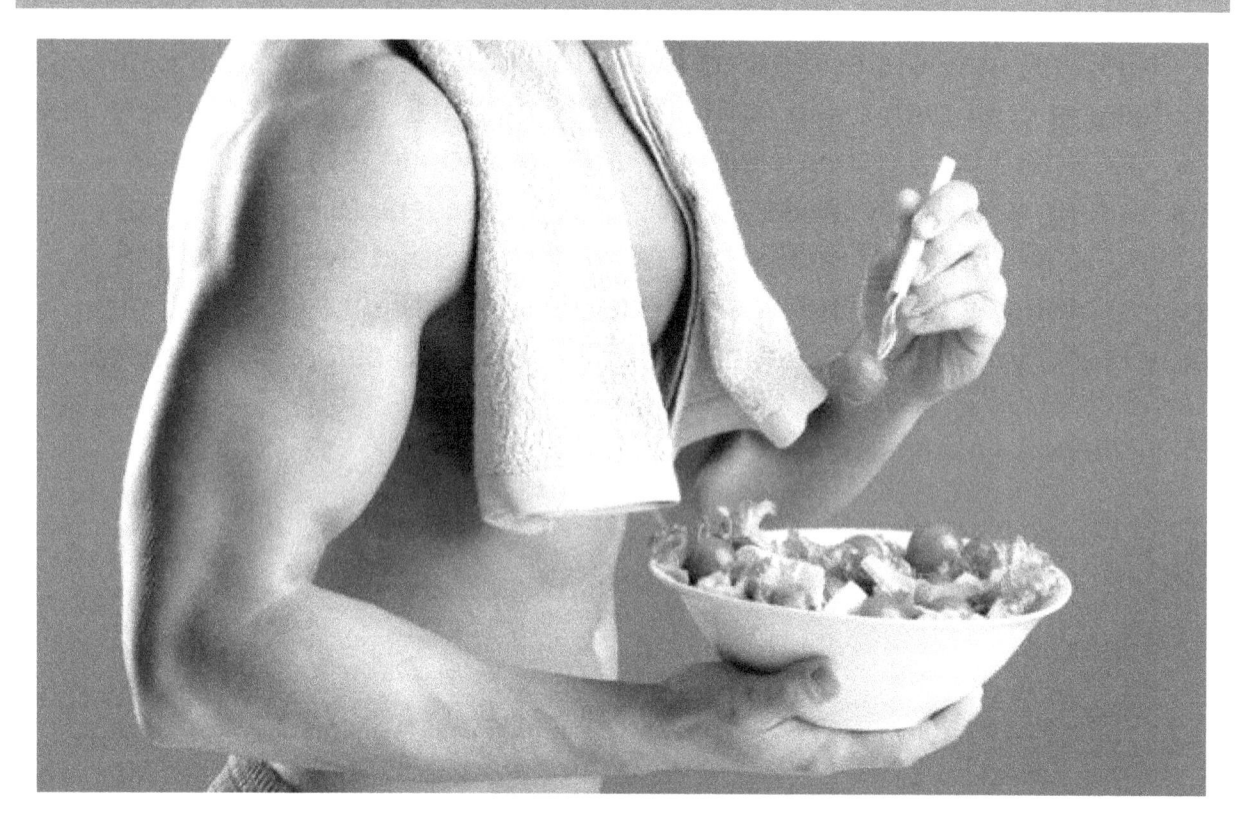

A balanced and proper diet is the key to good health and, if you want to gain muscle mass, it is the key to success. To do this, you need to include not only protein but also fats and carbohydrates on your menu.

From the right menu, the vegetarian can achieve the right amount of protein for muscle growth. Its primary function is to maintain and build the body tissue. However, it should be remembered that muscles will not grow only due to excessive intake of protein. Fats are also necessary for proper muscle growth. And if there are no or not enough fats in the diet, this will also affect the appearance of the athlete, and their body will become flabby, their hair will fall out, and their muscle mass will become weak.

Carbohydrates are considered to be the primary source of energy used during high-intensity activities. Studies indicate that including carbohydrates in the diet promotes performance and endurance. Scientists have proven that muscle building does not require as much protein as carbohydrates. And, if there is a lack of carbohydrates in the diet, but a large amount of protein instead, the body will transform it into carbohydrates itself. Thus, the athlete will only harm his health.

The balanced concept of nutrition for a vegan bodybuilder involves not only adequate protein intake, calorie control, and fat dosage. This is a certain system in which success depends literally on everything: the frequency of food intake, the total amount of proteins and dietary supplements are taken, the amount of fluid consumed, the combination of products and many other factors.

From how rationally the bodybuilder himself will be able to organize his diet - from the number of meals to the amount of water drunk - its result directly depends on a number of factors. Success, in this case, is a derivative of an integrated approach, and not just the influence of protein, as the followers of meat-eating believe.

The number of meals should be increased to six a day. These should be five main meals, and one before bedtime. With this approach, the muscles will continuously receive the necessary components, which means it will be much easier to build muscle. Not feeling hungry and at the same time, not overeating - this is the golden balance that any bodybuilder wants to achieve. If you do not follow this advice, the body will experience stress and store excess fat.

MACRONUTRIENT RATIOS

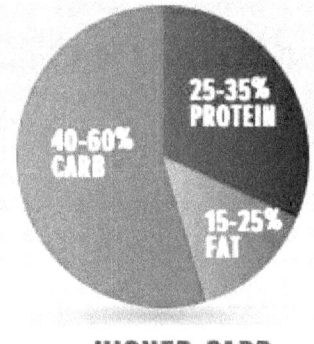

25-35% PROTEIN 40-60% CARB 15-25% FAT	25-35% PROTEIN 30-50% CARB 25-35% FAT	10-20% CARB 40-50% PROTEIN 30-40% FAT
HIGHER-CARB FOR BODYBUILDING	**MODERATE-CARB FOR MAINTENANCE**	**LOWER-CARB FOR FAT LOSS**

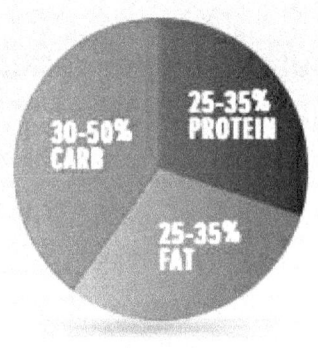

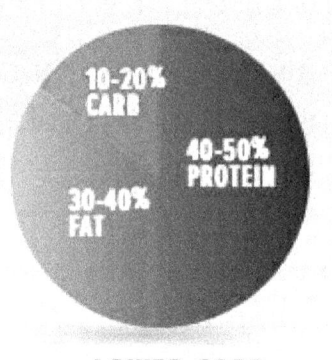

VEGAN COOKBOOK FOR BODYBUILDERS AND ATHLETES

EASY HIGH-PROTEIN PLANT-BASED RECIPES

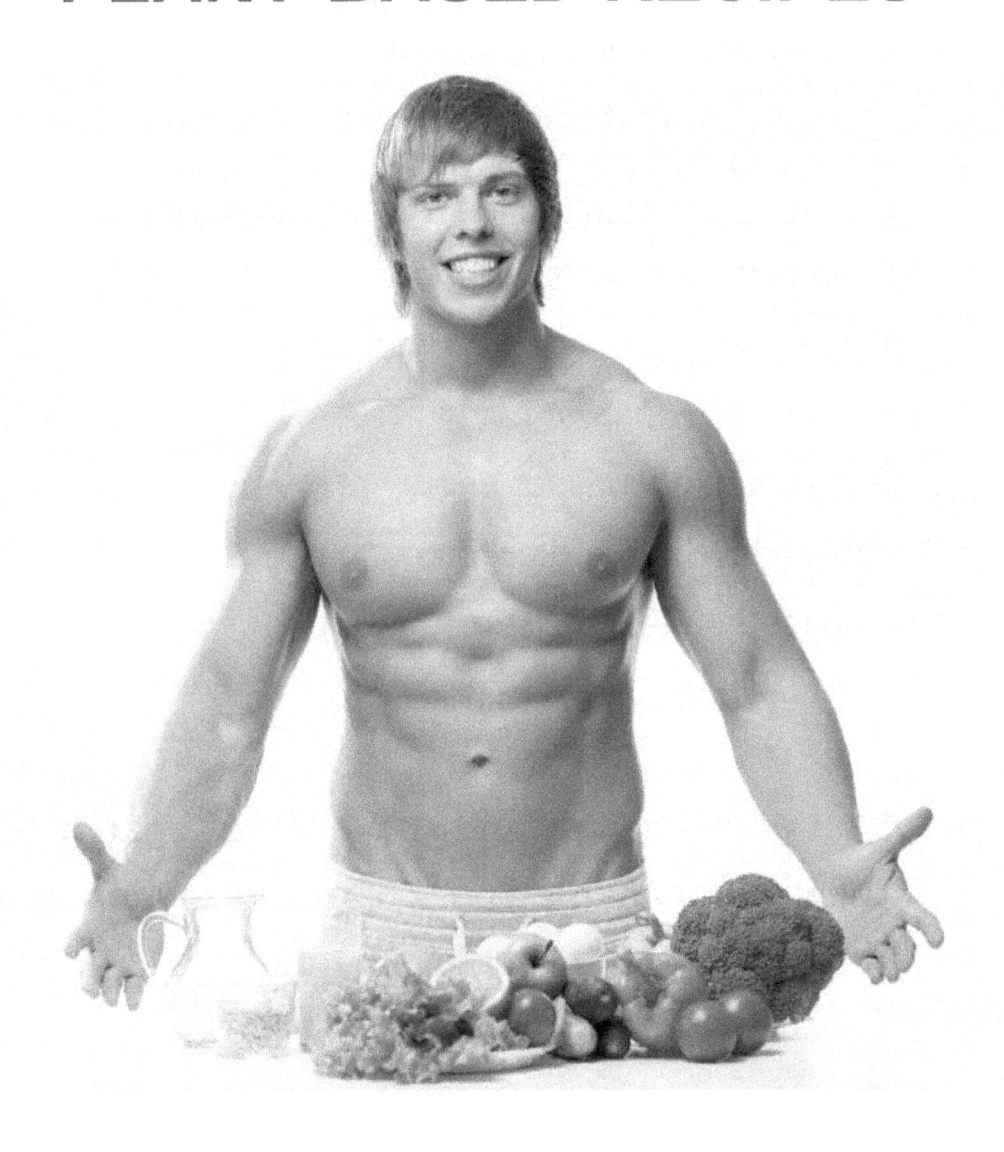

Vegetarian athletes, bodybuilders, fitness or sports enthusiast have special dietary needs.

In this recipe book, the author has collated the best high- protein no meat recipes designed specifically for vegetarian athletes who need to not only follow strict training rules but also want to eat something that tastes great.

This Vegan Cookbook contains high protein plant-based recipes optimized for athletes, bodybuilders, any fitness enthusiast, men and women for balanced athletic nutrition.

These easy-to-cook vegan recipes are suitable for anyone new to the vegan diet or cooking and will allow you to reduce your time in the kitchen in order to pay more attention to your workouts:

- High protein breakfasts for energy
- Protein salads with healthy nutrients
- First courses for proper nutrition
- Delicious staple foods for energy recovery
- Savory snacks and protein smoothies
- Plant-based protein desserts for a good

mood All recipes include full macro profiles.

Start cooking tasty and wholesome vegan food right now and recharge your batteries for your sporting achievements!

HIGH ENERGY BREAKFASTS

BLUEBERRY BANANA CHIA OATMEAL

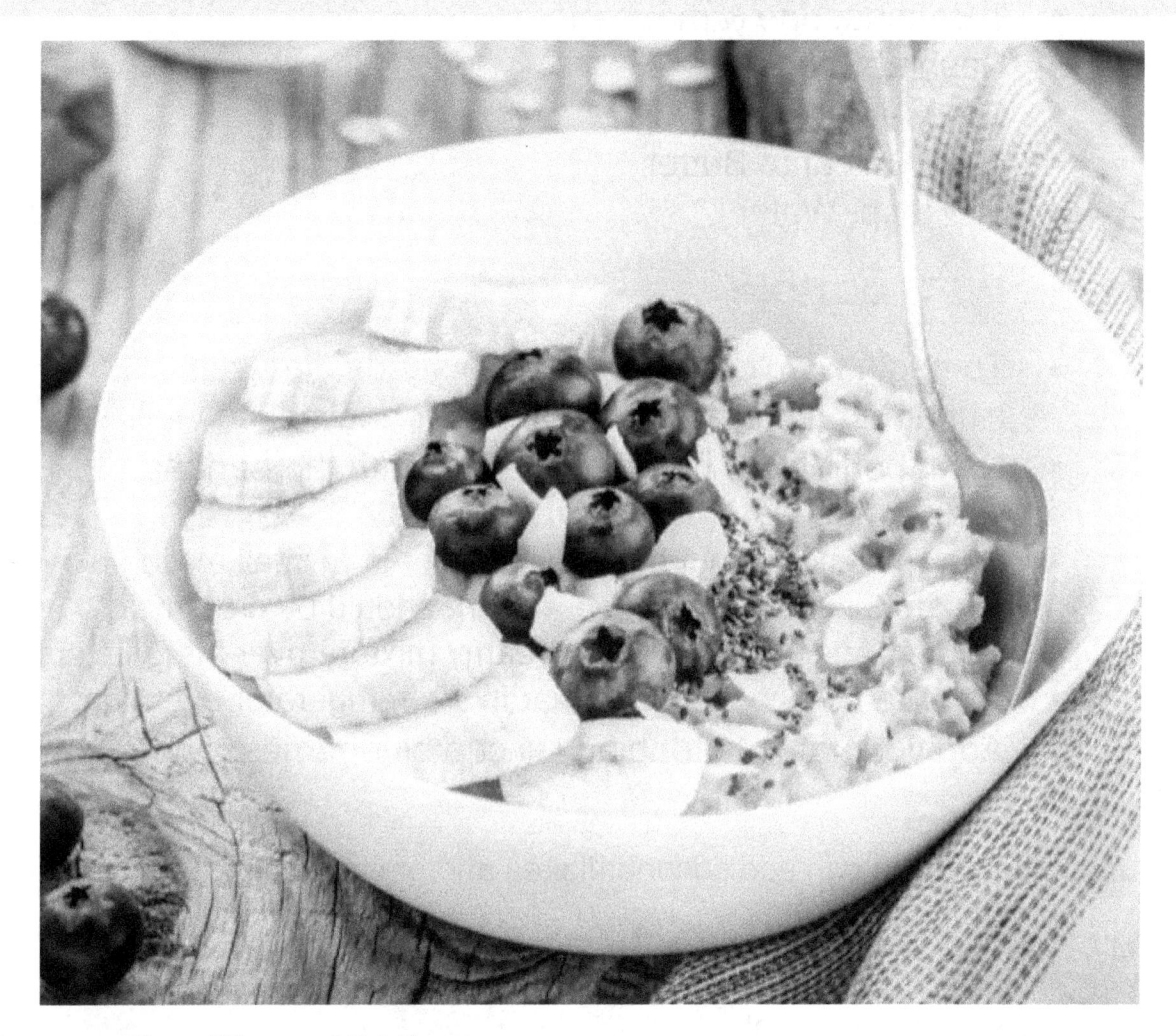

Preparation Time: 10 Minutes
Cooking Time: 10 Minutes
Skill: Beginner
Serving Size: 1

INGREDIENTS:

- ¾ cup Rolled Oats
- 1 cup Plant Milk
- 2 tbsp. Chia Seeds

- ¼ cup Blueberries
- ½ cup Water
- 2 tbsp. Agave Syrup
- ½ tsp. Cinnamon
- 1 Banana, ripe & mashed
- Dash of Sea Salt
- 1 tsp. Vanilla
- 2 tbsp. Peanut Butter
- 1 ½ tbsp. Water

COOKING INSTRUCTION:

- To begin with, combine the chia seeds, sea salt, cinnamon, and oats in a mason jar until mixed well.
- Next, pour in the hemp milk along with the banana, vanilla, and water to the jar. Stir again.
- Now, mix the peanut butter with water in a small mixing bowl for 2 to 3 minutes. Tip: The mixture should be creamy in
- texture. After that, pour the creamy mixture over the oats and
- stir. Then, place the mason jar in the refrigerator overnight.
- Add your favorite topping (¼ cup blueberries) and enjoy.

Tip: If you desire you can add coconut flakes and or cacao nibs as a topping.

NUTRITIONAL INFORMATION PER SERVING:

- Calories: 864Kcal
- Protein: 23g
- Carbohydrates: 107.4g
- Fat: 42.1g

BANANA STRAWBERRY OATS

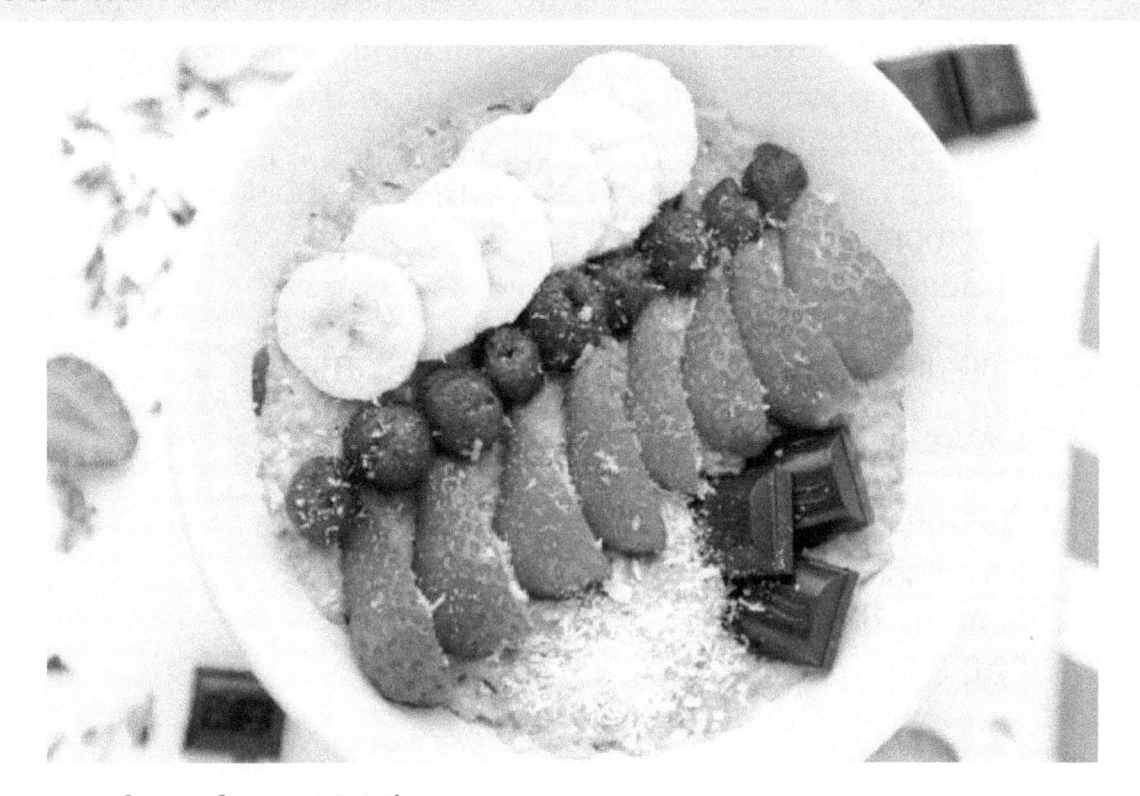

Preparation Time: 10 Minutes
Cooking Time: 20 Minutes
Skill: Beginner
Serving Size: 1

INGREDIENTS:

- ½ cup Oats
- 1 cup Zucchini, shredded
- 1 tbsp. Almonds, sliced
- ½ tsp. Cinnamon
- ½ of 1 Banana, mashed
- 1 cup Water
- ½ cup Strawberries, sliced
- Dash of Sea Salt
- 1 tbsp. Flax Meal
- ½ scoop of Protein Powder

COOKING INSTRUCTIONS:

- First, combine oats, salt, water, and zucchini in a large
- saucepan. Cook the mixture over medium-high heat and cook for 8 to 10 minutes or until the liquid is absorbed.
- Now, spoon in all the remaining ingredients to the mixture and give everything a good stir.
- Finally, transfer the mixture to a serving bowl and top it with almonds and berries.
- Serve and enjoy.

Tip: You can use any berries instead of strawberries.

NUTRITIONAL INFORMATION PER SERVING:

- Calories: 386Kcal
- Proteins: 23.7g
- Carbohydrates: 57.5g
- Fat: 8.9g

AVOCADO SWEET POTATO TOAST

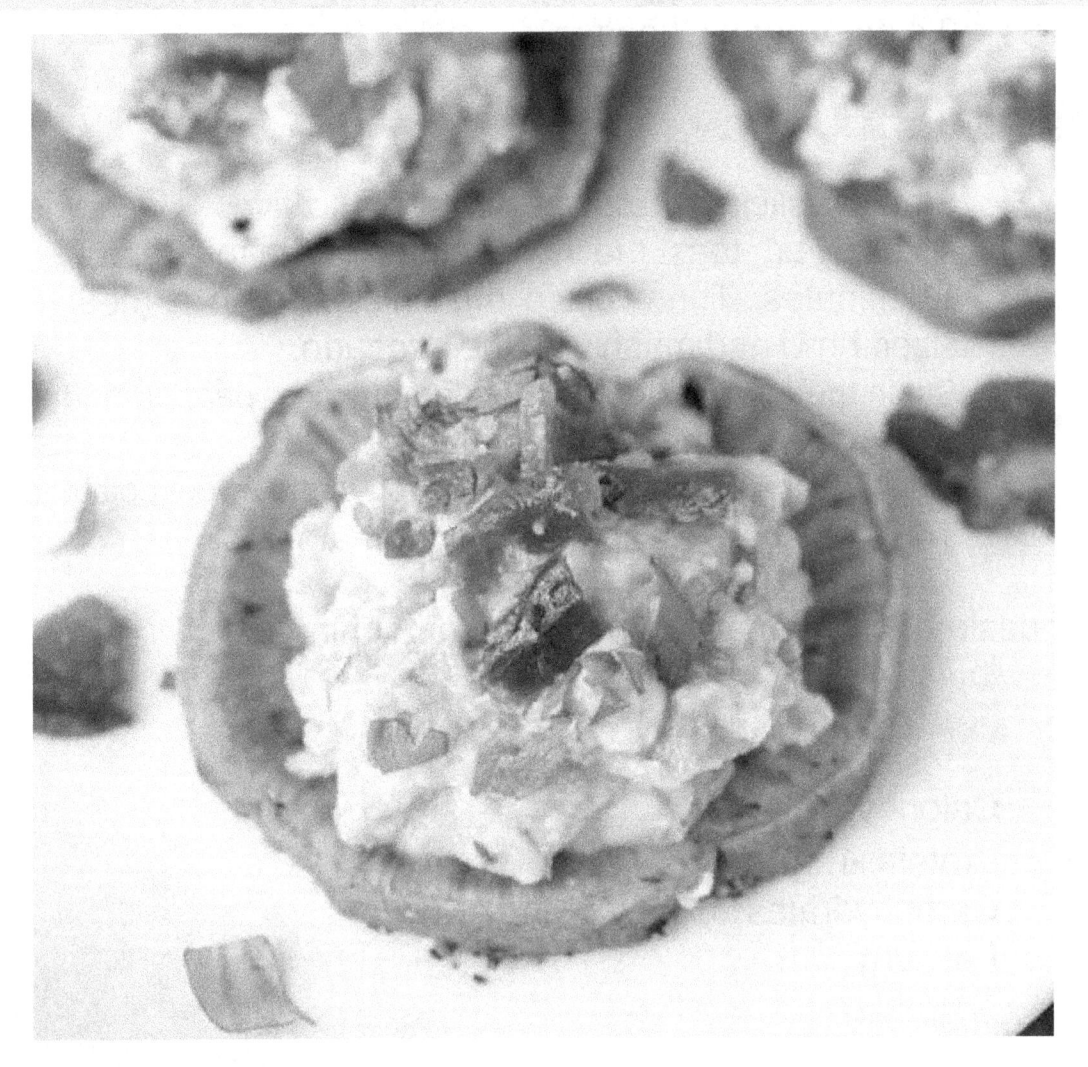

Preparation Time: 5 Minutes
Cooking Time: 10 Minutes
Skill: Beginner
Serving Size: 1

INGREDIENTS:

- 1 Sweet Potato, sliced into ¼-inch thick slices
- ½ of 1 Avocado, ripe
- ½ cup Chickpeas
- 2 tbsp. Sun-dried Tomatoes
- Salt & Pepper, as needed

- 1 tsp. Lemon Juice
- Pinch of Red Pepper
- 2 tbsp. Vegan Cheese

COOKING INSTRUCTION:

- Start by slicing the sweet potato into five ¼ inch wide
- slices. Next, toast the sweet potato in the toaster for 9 to
- 11 minutes. Then, place the chickpeas in a medium-sized bowl and mash with the avocado.
- Stir in the crushed red pepper, lemon juice, pepper, and salt.
- Stir until everything comes together.
- Finally, place the mixture on to the top of the sweet potato toast.
- Top with cheese and sun-dried tomatoes.

Tip: If desired, you can add your choice of toppings.

NUTRITIONAL INFORMATION PER SERVING:

- Calories: 452 Kcal
- Protein: 19g
- Carbohydrates: 77g
- Fat: 11g

BANANA QUINOA OATMEAL

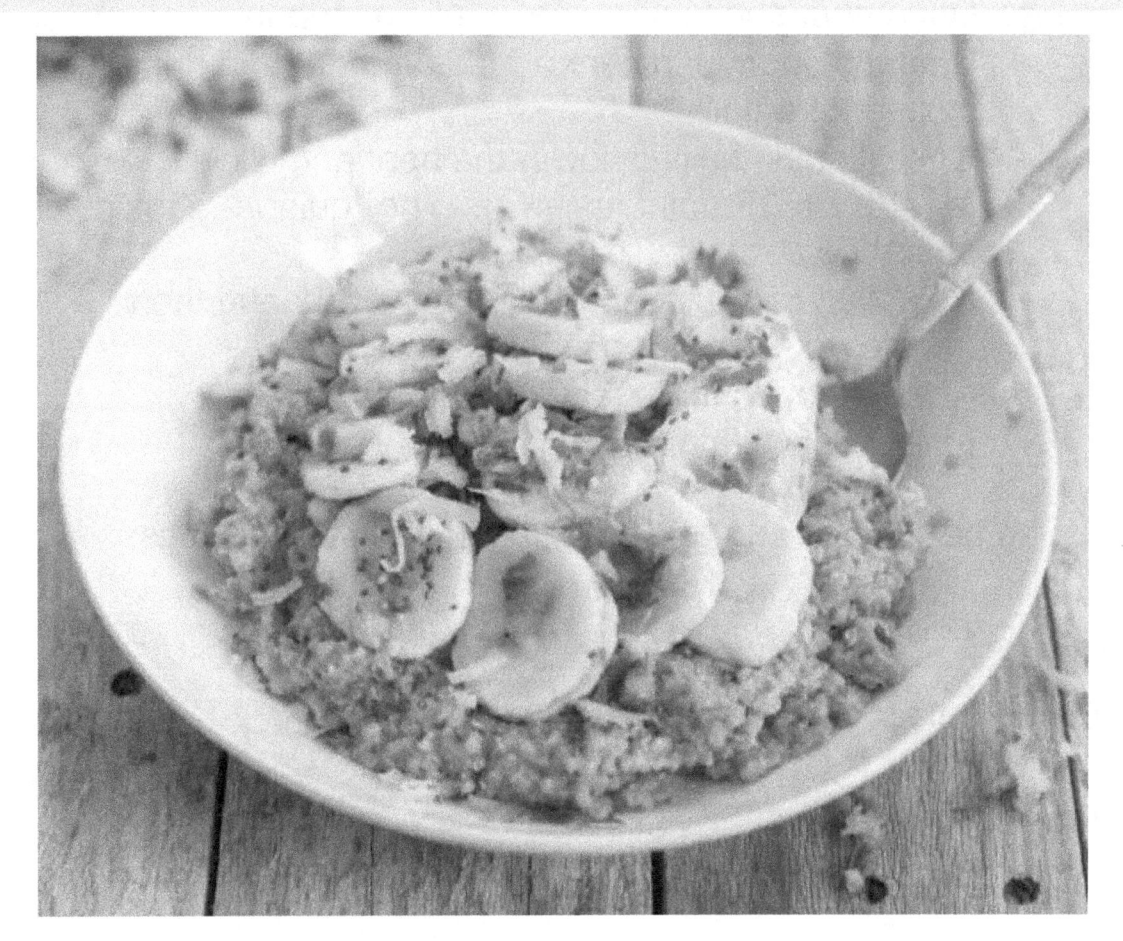

Preparation Time: 5 Minutes
Cooking Time: 10 Minutes
Skill: Beginner
Serving Size: 1

INGREDIENTS:

- ½ cup Oats
- ½ cup Quinoa, dry
- 2 Bananas, ripe
- ¾ cup Almond Milk, light
- ½ tsp. Cinnamon, ground
- 2 tbsp. Peanut Butter, organic
- 1 tsp. Vanilla

COOKING INSTRUCTION:

- To start, place the quinoa, nutmeg, almond milk, cinnamon, and vanilla in a small saucepan.
- Heat the saucepan over a medium heat and bring the mixture to a boil.
- Once it starts boiling, lower the heat and allow it to simmer for 10 to 15 minutes. Tip: The quinoa should have absorbed all the liquid in this time.
- Next, fluff the quinoa mixture with a fork and then transfer to a serving bowl.
- Now, spoon in the peanut butter and stir well.
- Finally, top with the banana.

Tip: If you desire, you can add almonds to it for crunchiness.

NUTRITIONAL INFORMATION PER SERVING:

- Calories: 386Kcal
- Protein: 11.7g
- Carbohydrates: 62.2g
- Fat: 11.8g

SPINACH TOFU SCRAMBLE

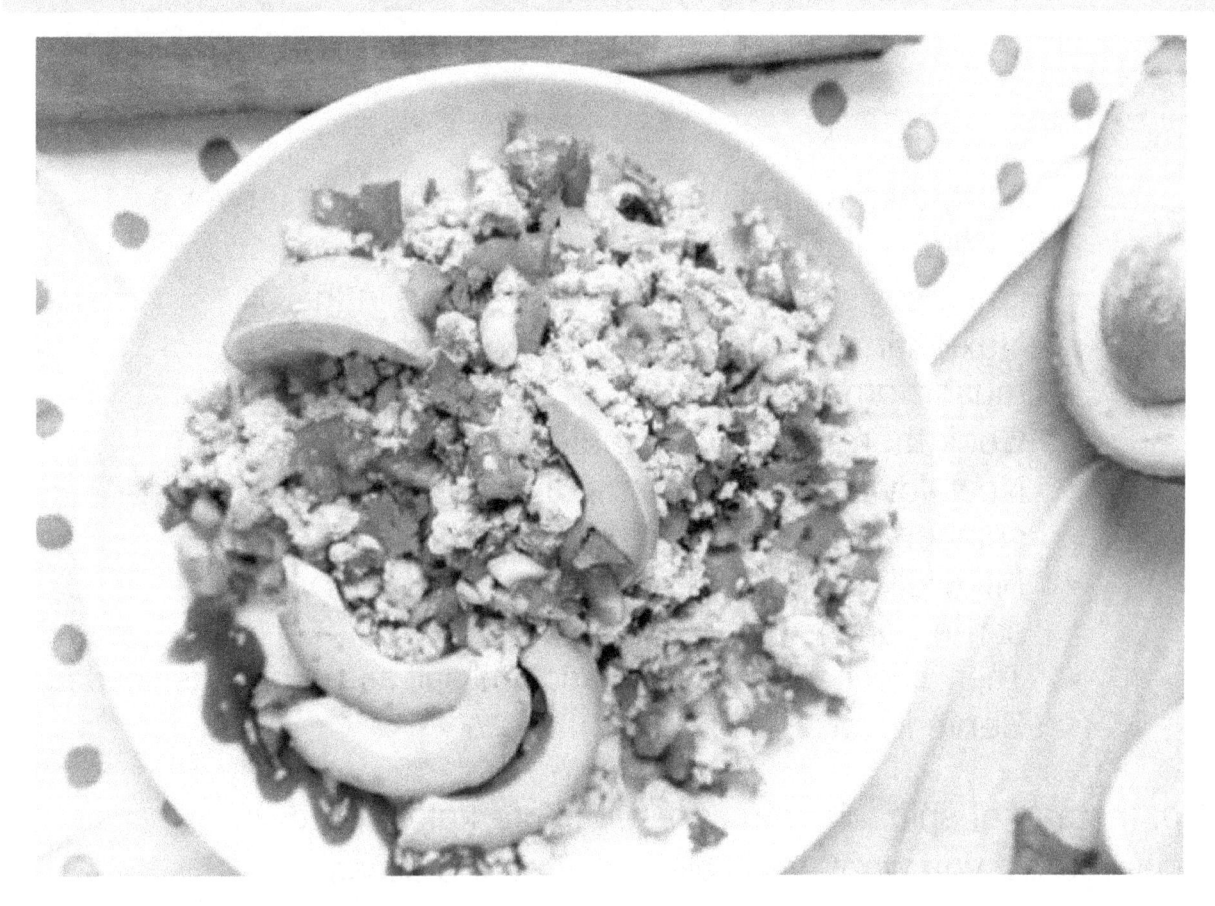

Preparation Time: 5 Minutes
Cooking Time: 10 Minutes
Skill: Beginner
Serving Size: 2

INGREDIENTS:

- 2 Tomatoes, finely chopped
- ¾ cup Mushrooms, finely sliced
- ½ red bell pepper, finely chopped
- 10 oz. Spinach
- 2 tbsp. Olive Oil
- 1 tsp. Lemon Juice, freshly squeezed
- ½ tsp. Soy Sauce
- 2 Garlic cloves, minced
- Salt & Pepper, as needed

- 1 lb. Tofu, extra-firm & crumbled
- 1 avocado (optional)

COOKING INSTRUCTION:

- First, take a medium-sized skillet and heat it over a medium-high heat.
- Once the skillet becomes hot, spoon in the oil.
- Next, stir in the tomatoes, red bell pepper, mushrooms, and garlic.
- Cook them for 2 to 3 minutes or until softened.
- Now, lower the heat to medium-low and spoon in the spinach, lemon juice, tofu, and soy sauce.
- Mix well and cook for a further 8 minutes while stirring occasionally.
- Then, check the seasoning and add salt and pepper as needed.
- Serve it hot.

Tip: Instead of spinach, you can substitute kale, chard, or asparagus. If you want, you can add avocado slices.

NUTRITIONAL INFORMATION PER SERVING:

- Calories: 527 Kcal
- Protein: 36g
- Carbohydrates: 43g
- Fat: 29g

HEMP SEEDS OATMEAL

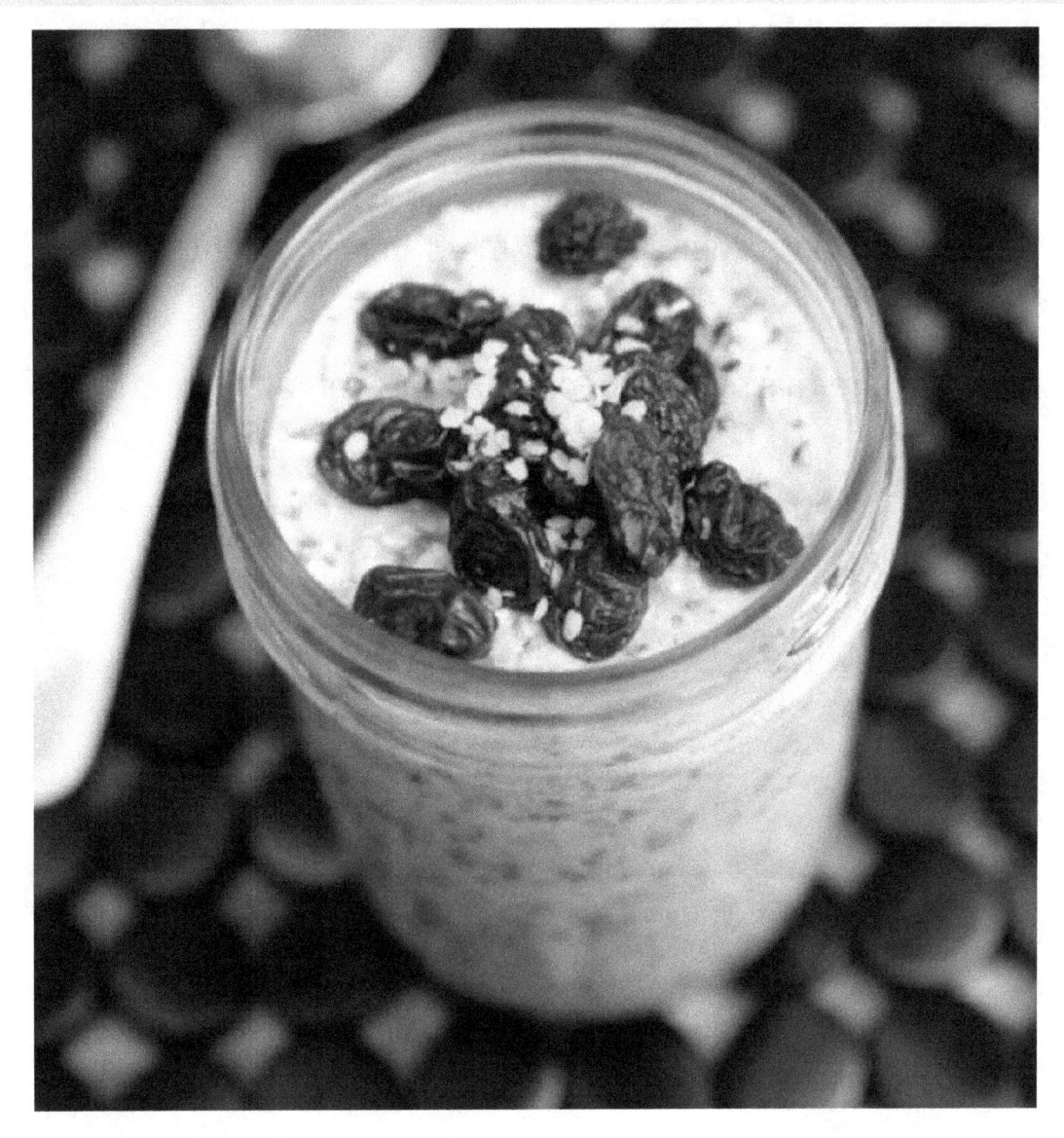

Preparation Time: 10 Minutes
Setting Time: 4 to 6 Hours
Skill: Beginner
Serving Size: 1

INGREDIENTS:

- ¼ cup Rolled Oats
- 1 tbsp. Raisins
- ¼ tsp. Cinnamon

- 3 tbsp. Hemp Seeds
- ½ cup Soy Milk, unsweetened
- 1 tbsp. Maple Syrup

COOKING INSTRUCTION:

- First, add all the ingredients to a large mason jar and mix well.
- Now, place them in the refrigerator overnight.
- Serve in the morning and enjoy.

Tip: To soften the raisins, you can soak them for a few hours.

NUTRITIONAL INFORMATION PER SERVING:

- Calories: 364 Kcal
- Protein: 19.1g
- Carbohydrates: 32.6g
- Fat: 19g

CHOCOLATE BREAKFAST QUINOA

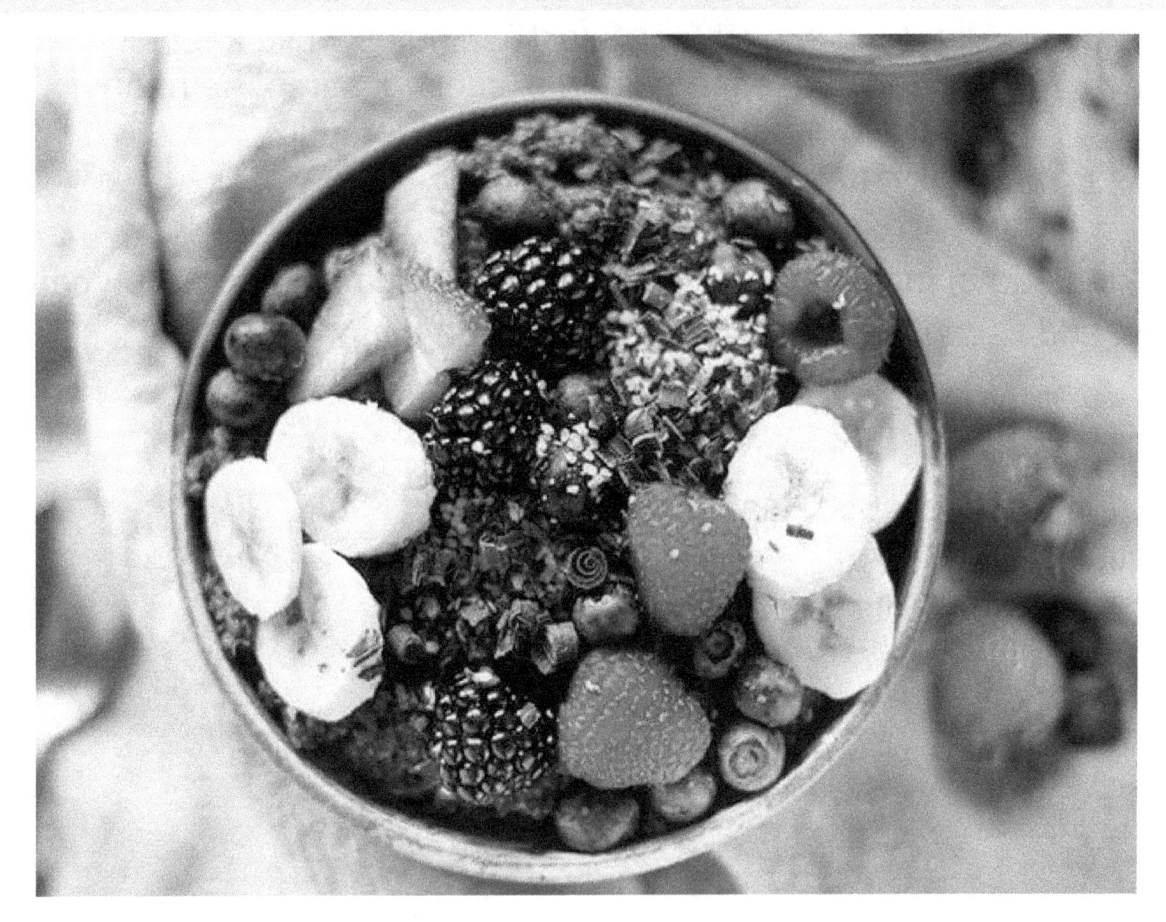

Preparation Time: 5 Minutes
Cooking Time: 20 Minutes
Skill: Beginner
Serving Size: 1

INGREDIENTS:

- ½ cup Quinoa
- 1 ½ tbsp. Cocoa
- 1 ½ cup Soy Milk
- 1 ½ tbsp. Maple Syrup
- 2 tbsp. Peanut Butter
- Banana and strawberry slices (for topping)

COOKING INSTRUCTION:

- First, place the quinoa and soy milk into a medium-sized saucepan over a medium-low heat.
- After that, cook it for 13 to 15 minutes while keeping it
- covered. Once the quinoa is cooked, stir in the peanut butter, sweetener, and cocoa powder to it.
- Finally, transfer to a serving bowl.

Tip: Instead of maple syrup, you can use brown rice syrup. You can even add cacao nibs to it. Also, you can add top any berries.

NUTRITIONAL INFORMATION PER SERVING:

- Calories: 650 Kcal
- Protein: 19g
- Carbohydrates: 97g
- Fat: 22g

BANANA CAULIFLOWER PORRIDGE

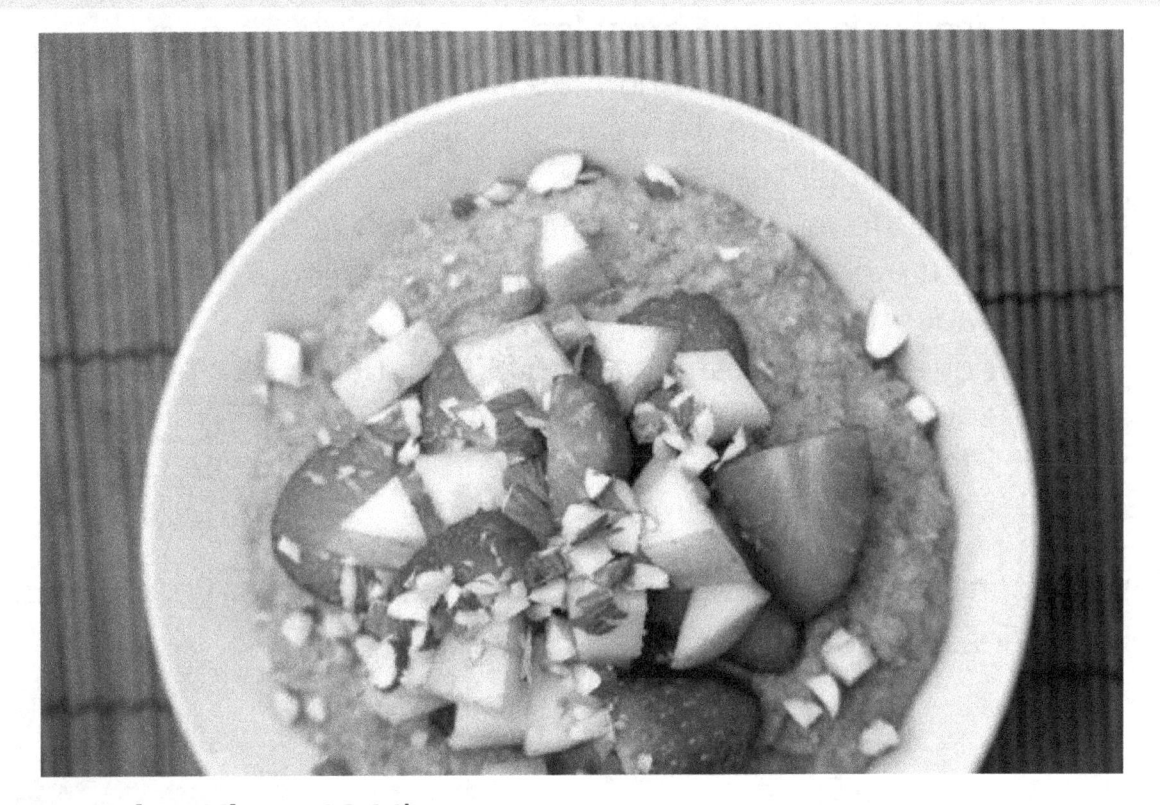

Preparation Time: 10 Minutes
Cooking Time: 15 Minutes
Skill: Beginner
Serving Size: 1

INGREDIENTS:

- 2 cups Cauliflower Extract
- ¼ of 1 Pear
- ½ of 1 Banana, ripe
- 1 cup Soy Milk, unsweetened
- ½ tsp. Vanilla Extract
- 1 ¼ tsp. Cinnamon
- 4 Strawberries
- 2 tsp. Maple Syrup
- ½ tbsp. Almond Butter
- 1/8 tsp. Salt

COOKING INSTRUCTION:

- To make this nutritious oatmeal, place the cauliflower in the food processor and process until the cauliflower becomes riced or is in small granules.
- Stir in the banana and mash it well.
- After that, place the riced cauliflower- banana mixture into a small saucepan.
- Heat the mixture over a medium-high heat.
- Next, spoon in all the remaining ingredients into the saucepan and give a good stir.
- Lower the heat and cook for 14 minutes. Continue cooking until ready.
- Place the oatmeal into a serving bowl and serve it immediately or warm.

Tip: You can even add sliced almonds to the mixture, or you can top it with berries and seeds.

NUTRITIONAL INFORMATION PER SERVING:

- Calories: 351 Kcal
- Protein: 15.1g
- Carbohydrates: 50.3g
- Fat: 12.1g

CHAI FLAVOURED QUINOA

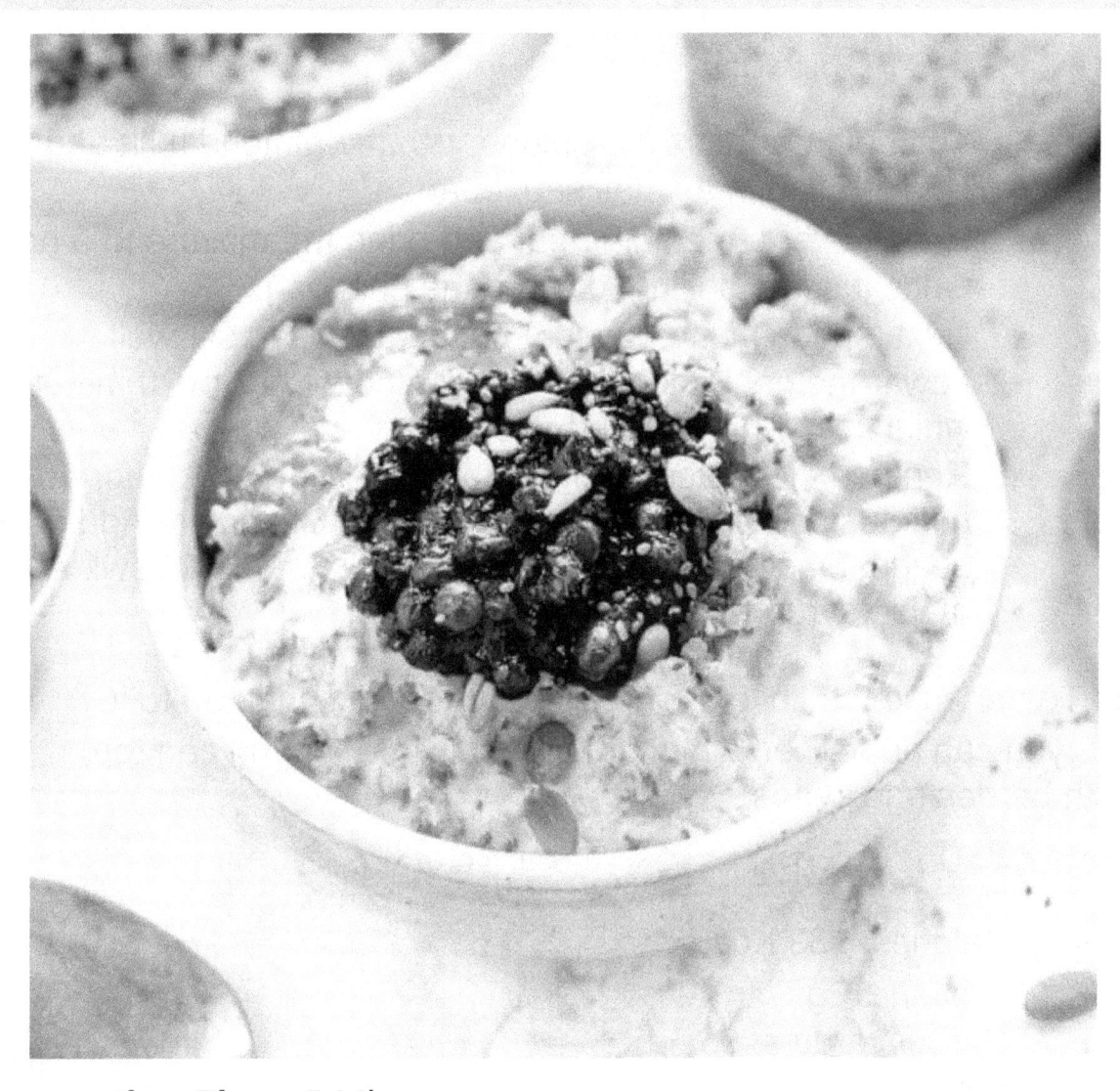

Preparation Time: 5 Minutes
Cooking Time: 20 Minutes
Skill: Beginner
Serving Size: 1

INGREDIENTS:

- ½ cup Quinoa, washed
- ½ tbsp. Coconut Palm Sugar
- 2 tbsp. Chia Seeds
- 2 tsp. Maple Syrup

- 1 Chai Tea Bag
- 1 cup Almond Milk, unsweetened

COOKING INSTRUCTION:

- To begin with, mix the quinoa with the almond milk and chai tea bag in a small saucepan.
- Heat it over a medium heat and bring the mixture to a boil.
- Once it starts boiling, discard the chai bag.
- Next, spoon in the coconut palm sugar and stir well.
- Lower the heat and allow it to simmer for 18 to 20 minutes while keeping it covered.
- Remove the saucepan from the heat. Set it aside for 10 minutes so that the quinoa absorbs all the liquid. Add chia
- seeds. Finally, transfer the mixture to a serving bowl. Add
- maple syrup. Serve immediately.

Tip: To enhance the flavor, you can add ground cinnamon to it. Also, you can add sliced almonds to the mixture, or you can top it with berries and seeds.

NUTRITIONAL INFORMATION PER SERVING:

- Calories: 383 Kcal
- Protein: 13g
- Carbohydrates: 65.6g
- Fat: 8.7g

PROTEIN SALAD

PEANUT NOODLE SALAD

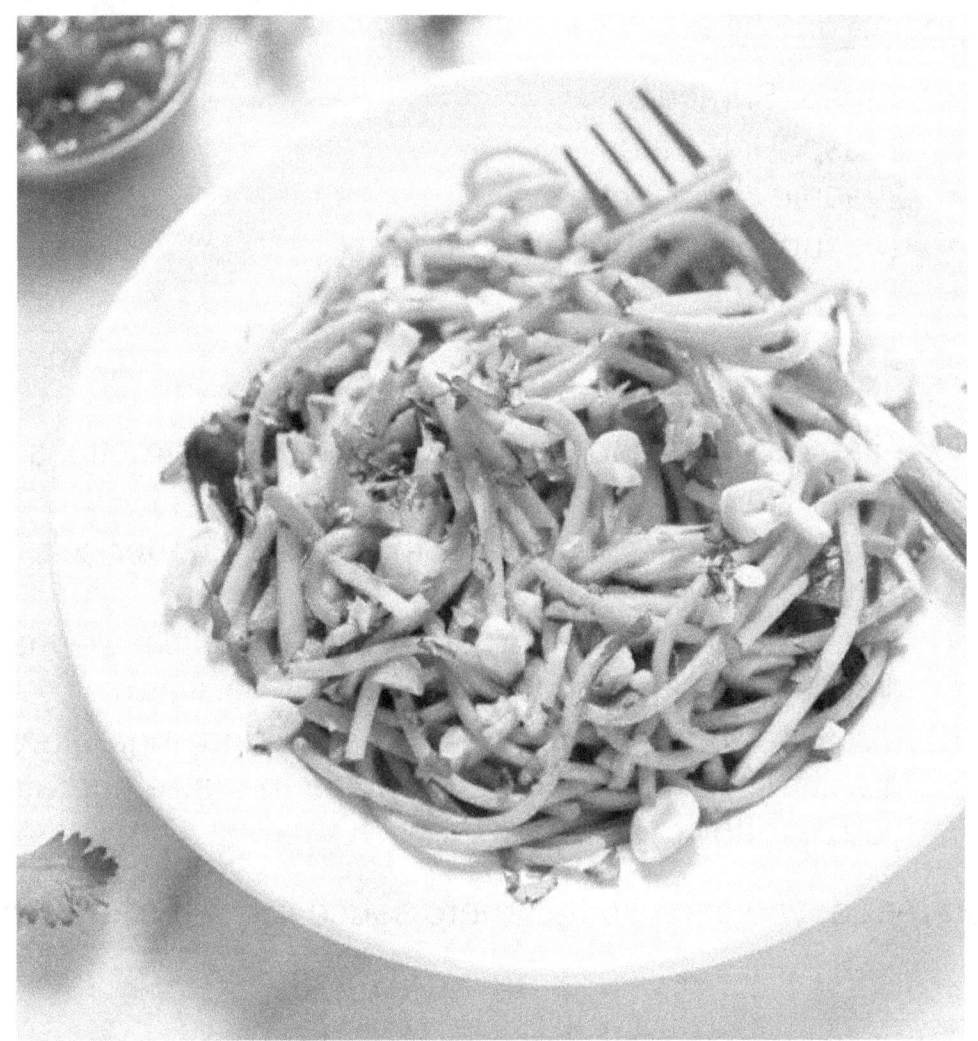

Preparation Time: 20 Minutes
Cooking Time: 5 Minutes
Skill: Beginner
Serving Size: 2

INGREDIENTS:

For the salad:

- 1 cup Carrots, shredded
- 1/3 cup Peanuts, chopped

- 8 oz. Rice Noodles
- ½ of 1 Red Bell Pepper, sliced thinly
- 2 Scallions, chopped
- ½ tsp. Black Sesame Seeds

For the peanut dressing:

- 3 tbsp. Sriracha
- 2 tbsp. Hot Water
- 2 Garlic cloves, minced
- 1/3 cup Peanut Butter, creamy
- 1 tbsp. Rice Vinegar

COOKING INSTRUCTION:

- First, cook the noodles by following the instructions given on the packet.
- Drain the excess water and then rinse it under cold water. Keep aside.
- After that, combine all the ingredients needed to make the dressing in a small bowl until mixed well. Set it aside.
- Mix the noodles with all the remaining ingredients and
- dressing. Combine and then place in the refrigerator until you're ready to serve.

Tip: If preferred, you can use habanero sauce instead of sriracha.

NUTRITIONAL INFORMATION PER SERVING:

- Calories: 604 Kcal
- Protein: 25g
- Carbohydrates: 90g
- Fat: 17g

BROCCOLI EDAMAME SALAD

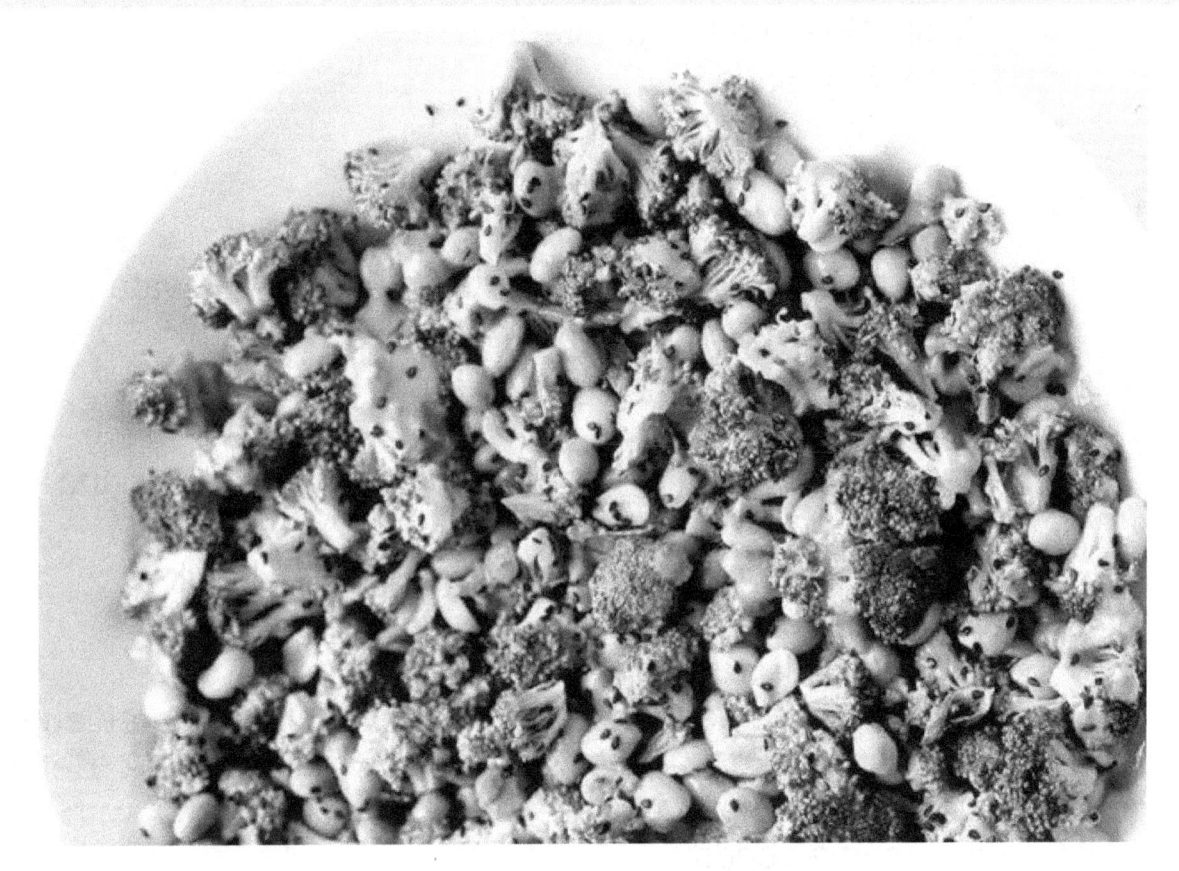

Preparation Time: 10 Minutes
Cooking Time: 20 Minutes
Skill: Beginner
Serving Size: 4 to 6

INGREDIENTS:

For the salad:

- 1 Broccoli head, large & torn into florets
- 1 cup Edamame, shelled & cooked
- ½ cup Peanuts
- Sesame Seeds, as needed, for garnishing
- ½ cup Green onion, sliced thinly

For the peanut sauce:

- 1 tbsp. Rice Vinegar

- 2 tbsp. Hot Water
- ¼ cup Peanut Butter, natural
- 1/8 tsp. Sesame Oil, toasted
- 1 tbsp. Soy Sauce
- 1 tbsp. Agave Nectar

COOKING INSTRUCTION:

- To make this easy salad, you first need to heat water in a large pot over medium heat.
- Once it starts boiling, stir in the broccoli and cook for half a minute.
- After that, transfer the cooked broccoli to a strainer and place in a bowl of cold water.
- Drain the broccoli and put in a large mixing bowl.
- Add all the remaining salad ingredients to the bowl and toss well.
- Now, make the peanut sauce by mixing all the ingredients needed to make the dressing in a bowl with a whisk. Set it
- aside. Finally, spoon in the dressing and garnish it with the sesame seeds.

Tip: Instead of soy sauce, you can also use tamari.

NUTRITIONAL INFORMATION PER SERVING:

- Calories: 543 Kcal
- Protein: 36g
- Carbohydrates: 85.4g
- Fat: 36g

BLACK BEAN LENTIL SALAD

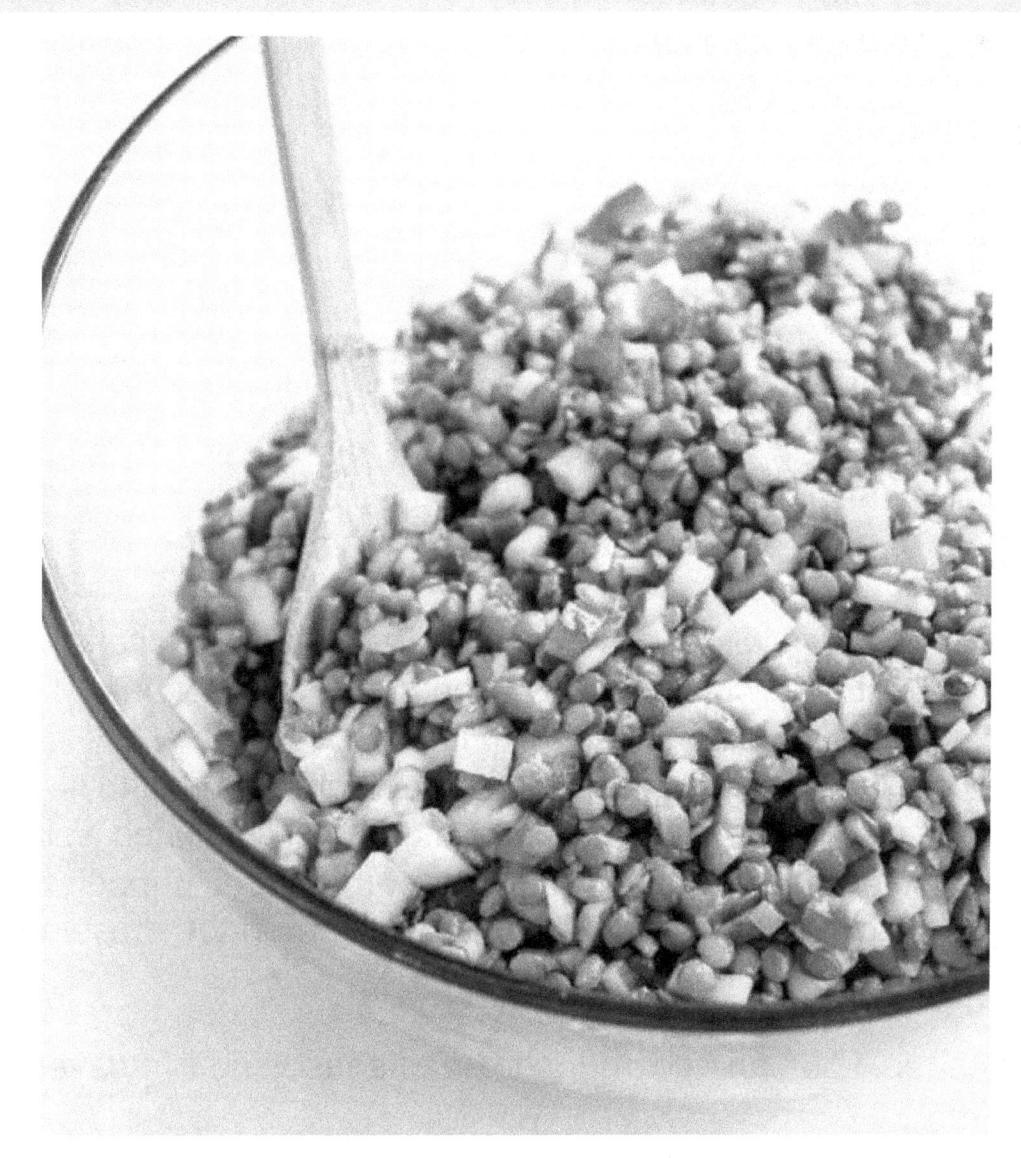

Preparation Time: 10 Minutes
Cooking Time: 20 Minutes
Skill: Beginner
Serving Size: 5

INGREDIENTS:

- 1 Red Bell Pepper, diced
- 1 Cucumber, diced
- ½ of 1 Red Onion, small & diced
- 2/3 cup Cilantro

- 1 cup Green Lentils
- 2 Roma Tomatoes, diced
- 15 oz. Black Beans

For dressing:

- ½ tsp. Oregano
- Juice of 1 Lime
- 1/8 tsp. Salt
- 2 tbsp. Olive Oil
- 1 tsp. Cumin
- 1 tsp. Dijon Mustard
- 2 Garlic cloves

COOKING INSTRUCTION:

- To begin with, cook the lentils in a large pan over a medium heat following the manufacturer's instructions. Tip: The lentils should be cooked to firm but not mushy.
- In the meantime, mix all the ingredients needed to make the dressing in a small bowl until combined well.
- After that, combine the beans with the bell pepper, red onion cilantro, and cucumber. Spoon on the dressing.
- Toss well and serve immediately.

Tip: If desired, you can add your choice of seasoning like cayenne pepper, etc.

NUTRITIONAL INFORMATION PER SERVING:

- Calories: 285 Kcal
- Protein: 15g
- Carbohydrates: 41g
- Fat: 6g

TOMATO GREEN LENTIL SALAD

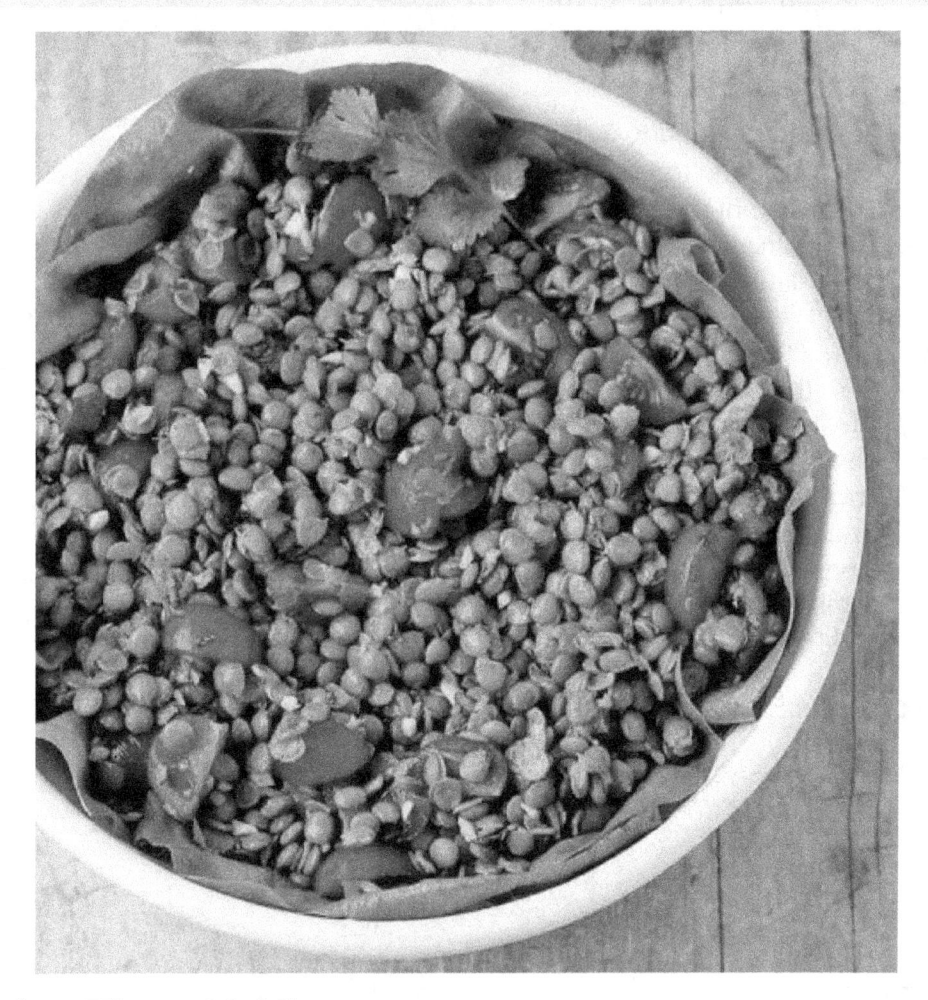

Preparation Time: 10 Minutes
Cooking Time: 30 Minutes
Skill: Beginner
Serving Size: 6

INGREDIENTS:

For the salad:

- 1 cup Green Lentil
- ½ cup Celery, diced
- 1 cup Red Onion, sliced
- 1 tbsp. Olive Oil, divided
- 2 tbsp. Extra Virgin Olive Oil
- ¼ tsp. Crushed Red Pepper
- 1 ½ cup Grape Tomatoes, halved
- 1 Head of Garlic
- 2 tbsp. Lemon Juice

- ½ cup Red Pepper, diced
- Salt & Pepper, as needed
- 2 ¾ cup Vegetable Broth

COOKING INSTRUCTION:

- Preheat the oven to 375 ° F.
- Next, slice the top of the garlic head and put in foil.
- Brush half of the olive oil on the garlic and close the foil.
- Then, place the tomatoes and onion in a single layer on a parchment paper-lined baking sheet.
- Spoon the olive oil over the tomato-onion mixture. Sprinkle salt and pepper over it.
- Now, cook for 28 to 30 minutes or until slightly dried.
- After that, open the foil and allow the garlic to cool.
- Take the garlic cloves from the head and keep in a bowl while breaking the garlic.
- Meanwhile, bring the broth mixture to a boil and stir in lentils to it.
- Lower the heat and simmer for 28 to 30 minutes or until tender.
- Drain the lentils and set aside.
- Meanwhile, whisk all the ingredients in a small bowl together until
- combined well. Finally, add the tomatoes, celery, red pepper, tomatoes, and red onion. Spoon the dressing and serve immediately.

Tip: Instead of roasted tomatoes, you can also use sun-dried tomatoes.

NUTRITIONAL INFORMATION PER SERVING:

- Calories: 194 Kcal
- Protein: 8g
- Carbohydrates: 23g
- Fat: 7g

ARUGULA GREEN BEANS SALAD

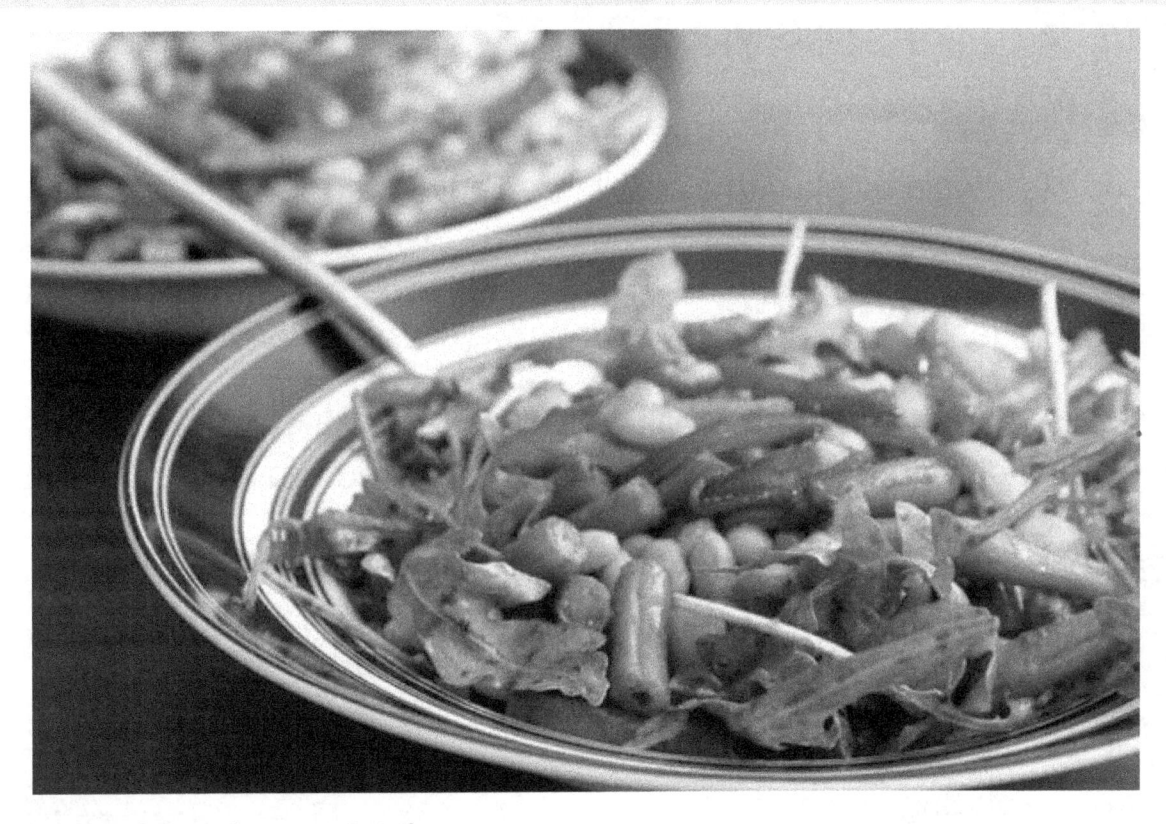

Preparation Time: 10 Minutes
Cooking Time: 25 Minutes
Skill: Beginner
Serving Size: 8

INGREDIENTS:

For the salad:

- 2 handful of Arugula
- 4 tbsp. Capers
- 15 oz. Lentils, cooked
- 15 oz. Green Kidney Beans

For the dressing:

- 1 tbsp. Balsamic Vinegar
- 1 tbsp. Tamari
- 2 tbsp. Peanut Butter

- 1 tbsp. Caper Brine
- 1 tbsp. Tahini
- 2 tbsp. Hot Sauce

COOKING INSTRUCTION:

- Begin by placing all the ingredients needed to make the dressing in a medium bowl and whisk it well until combined.
- After that, combine the arugula, capers, kidney beans, and lentils in a large bowl. Pour the dressing over it. Serve and
- enjoy.

Tip: Instead of green beans, you can also use red beans.

NUTRITIONAL INFORMATION PER SERVING:

- Calories: 543 Kcal
- Protein: 36g
- Carbohydrates: 85.4g
- Fat: 36g

SORGHUM KALE PESTO SALAD

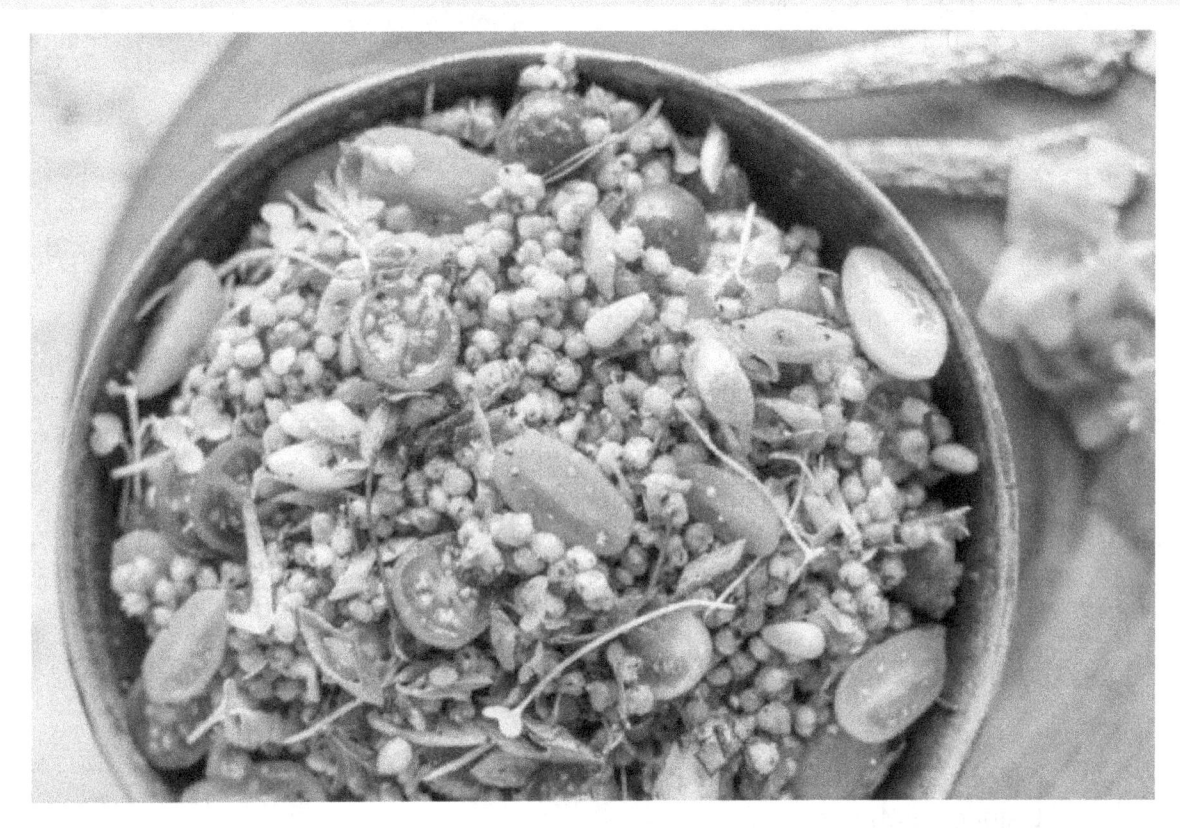

Preparation Time: 5 Minutes
Cooking Time: 55 Minutes
Skill: Beginner
Serving Size: 4

INGREDIENTS:

- 1 cup Sorghum
- 3 cups Water
- Dash of Salt

For the salad:

- 3 tbsp. Parsley, chopped
- 6 oz. Plum Tomatoes
- 1 Green Onion Stalk, sliced thinly
- Salt & Pepper, to taste
- Handful of Greens

For the pesto:

- 1 1/3 cup Kale leaves
- 1/3 cup Pine Nuts
- 1 Garlic Clove, large

- ¾ cup Basil, fresh
- ½ tbsp. Yellow Miso Paste
- 1 tbsp. Lemon Juice
- ¼ cup Olive Oil
- 3 tbsp. Water
- 3 tbsp. Nutritional Yeast

COOKING INSTRUCTION:

- To start with, place the sorghum, water, and salt in a large saucepan and heat it over a medium-high heat.
- Bring the mixture to a boil. Lower the heat.
- Cook the grains for 50 minutes keeping it half covered.
- When the grains become soft, yet chewy, remove the pan from the heat.
- Drain the water and then prepare the pesto by placing all the ingredients in the food processor.
- Blend it for 1 to 2 minutes or until the pesto is smooth.
- Next, combine the cooked sorghum with ¼ of the pesto in a large mixing bowl.
- Stir in the plum tomatoes, chopped parsley, greens, parsley, and nuts. Mix well.
- Taste for seasoning. Add more salt and pepper if needed.

Tip: If desired, you can add your choice of seasoning like cayenne pepper, etc.

NUTRITIONAL INFORMATION PER SERVING:

- Calories: 508 Kcal
- Protein: 13.1g
- Carbohydrates: 78.7g
- Fat: 18.8g

RED CABBAGE SALAD

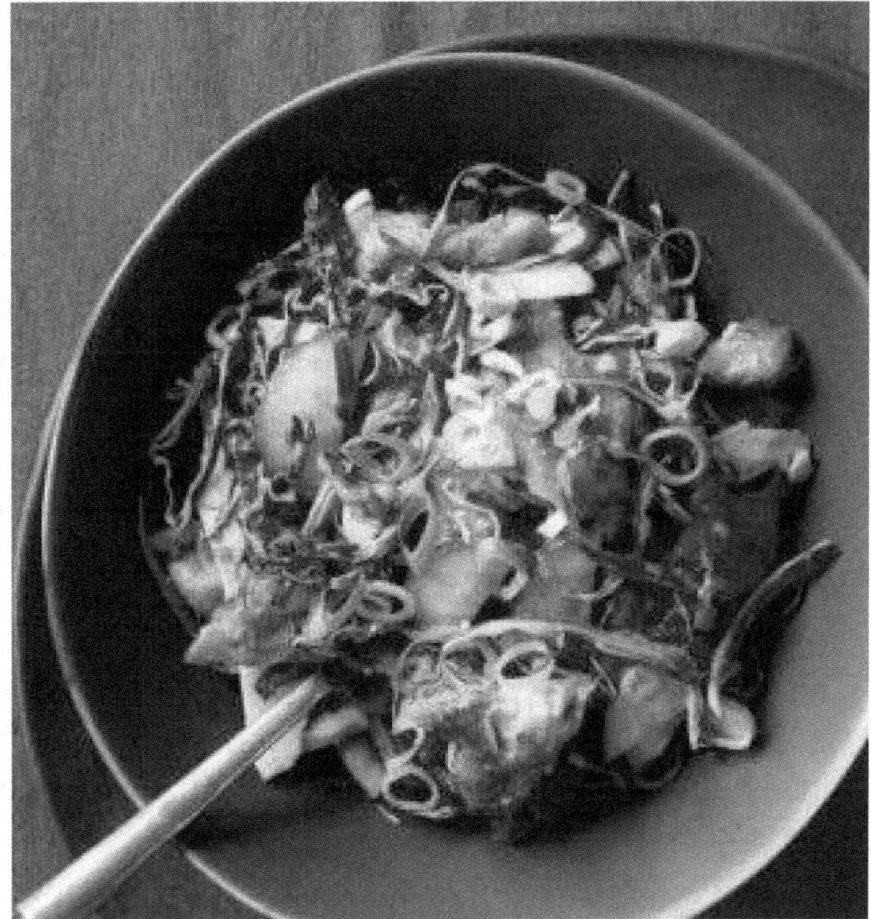

Preparation Time: 5 Minutes
Cooking Time: 55 Minutes
Skill: Beginner
Serving Size: 4

INGREDIENTS:

For the dressing:

- 1/3 cup Peanut Butter, natural &
- creamy 1/3 cup Mango Chutney

For the salad:

- 3 Green Onions, sliced thinly
- 1 Cucumber, small & cut into half thin moons

- 1 tbsp. Olive Oil
- 18 oz. Seitan, sliced into strips
- 3 Garlic Cloves, minced
- 6 cups Red Cabbage, shredded
- ¾ tsp. Curry Powder, mild

COOKING INSTRUCTION:

- First, to make the dressing you need to combine the chutney, 1/3 cup water, and peanut butter in a high-speed blender.
- Blend the mixture until it becomes smooth. Set the dressing aside.
- After that, take a large skillet and heat it over medium heat.
- Stir in one tablespoon of olive oil and then the seitan.
- Add salt if needed and sauté the seitan for 5 to 7 minutes or until it becomes brown.
- Next, spoon in the garlic and the remaining olive oil.
- Cook for a further 30 seconds and then add the curry powder.
- Sauté for 2 minutes and remove from the heat.
- Finally, add the cabbage and cucumber along with the dressing in a large mixing bowl.
- Top it with the seitan and green onions.
- Serve immediately.

Tip: If preferred, you can add carrots also.

NUTRITIONAL INFORMATION PER SERVING:

- Calories: 330 Kcal
- Protein: 15g
- Carbohydrates: 32g
- Fat: 19g

QUINOA CHICKPEAS AVOCADO SALAD

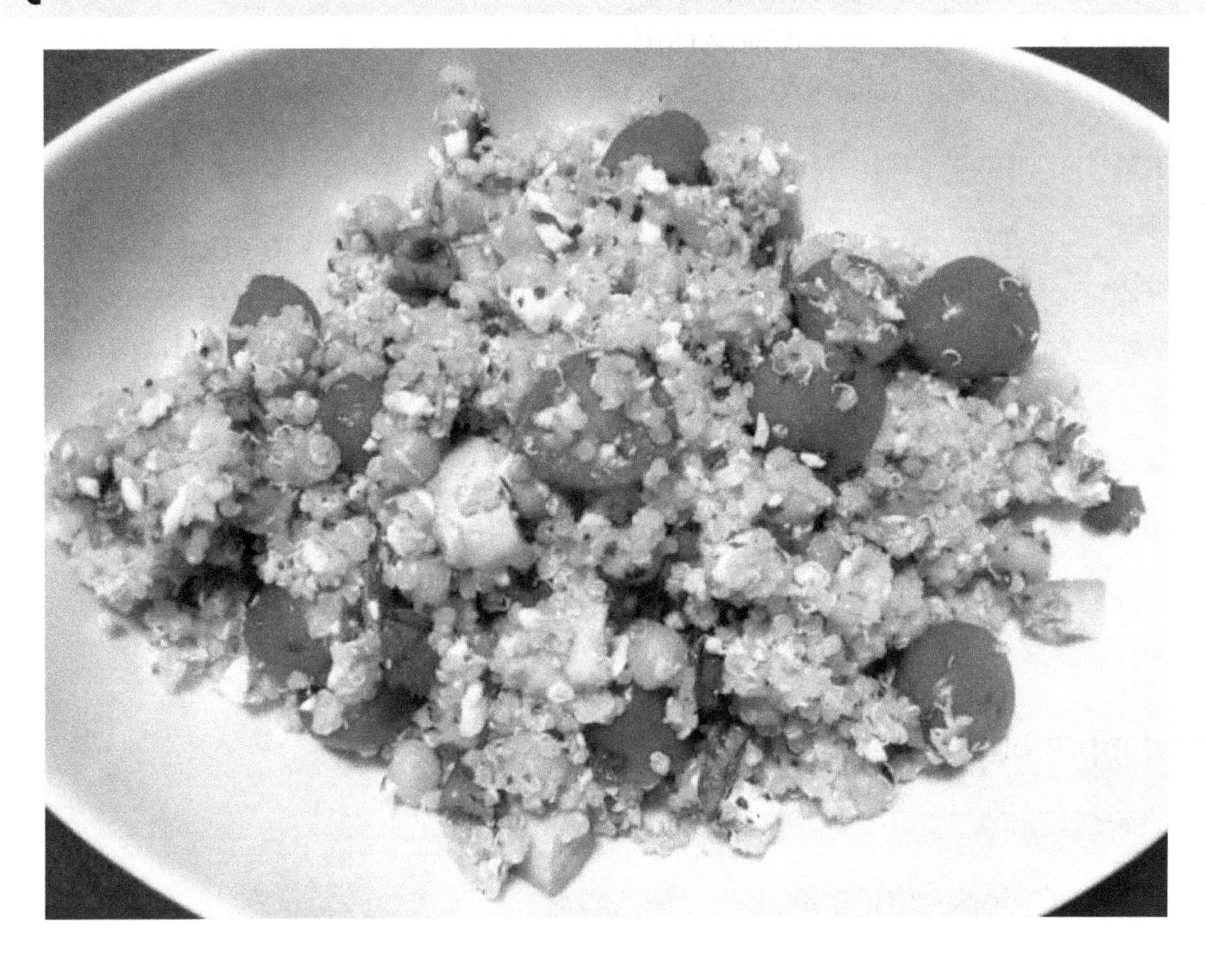

Preparation Time: 10 Minutes
Cooking Time: 20 Minutes
Skill: Beginner
Serving Size: 4

INGREDIENTS:

<u>For the salad:</u>

- 1 Avocado, medium & diced
- 1 ½ tbsp. Tahini
- 30 Cherry Tomatoes, sliced
- 4 ½ cups Chickpeas, cooked
- ¼ tsp. Salt
- ½ of 1 Red Onion, medium & diced
- 1/3 cup Water

- 2 tbsp. Lemon Juice
- Pepper, as needed
- 1 ½ tsp. Dijon Mustard
- ½ cup Cilantro, packed

COOKING INSTRUCTION:

- To make this healthy salad, you first need to cook the quinoa by following the instructions given on the packet.
- Next, take 1/3 rd of the chickpeas and place in a high-speed blender along with the water, lemon juice, pepper, Dijon mustard, and salt.
- Blend for a minute or until you get a creamy consistency.
- Now, toss the cooked quinoa, cherry tomatoes, red onion, avocado, and cilantro into a large mixing bowl. Drizzle the
- dressing over it and serve immediately.

Tip: If preferred, you can add carrots also.

NUTRITIONAL INFORMATION PER SERVING:

- Calories: 604 Kcal
- Protein: 25g
- Carbohydrates: 90g
- Fat: 17g

BUTTERNUT SQUASH SPINACH SALAD

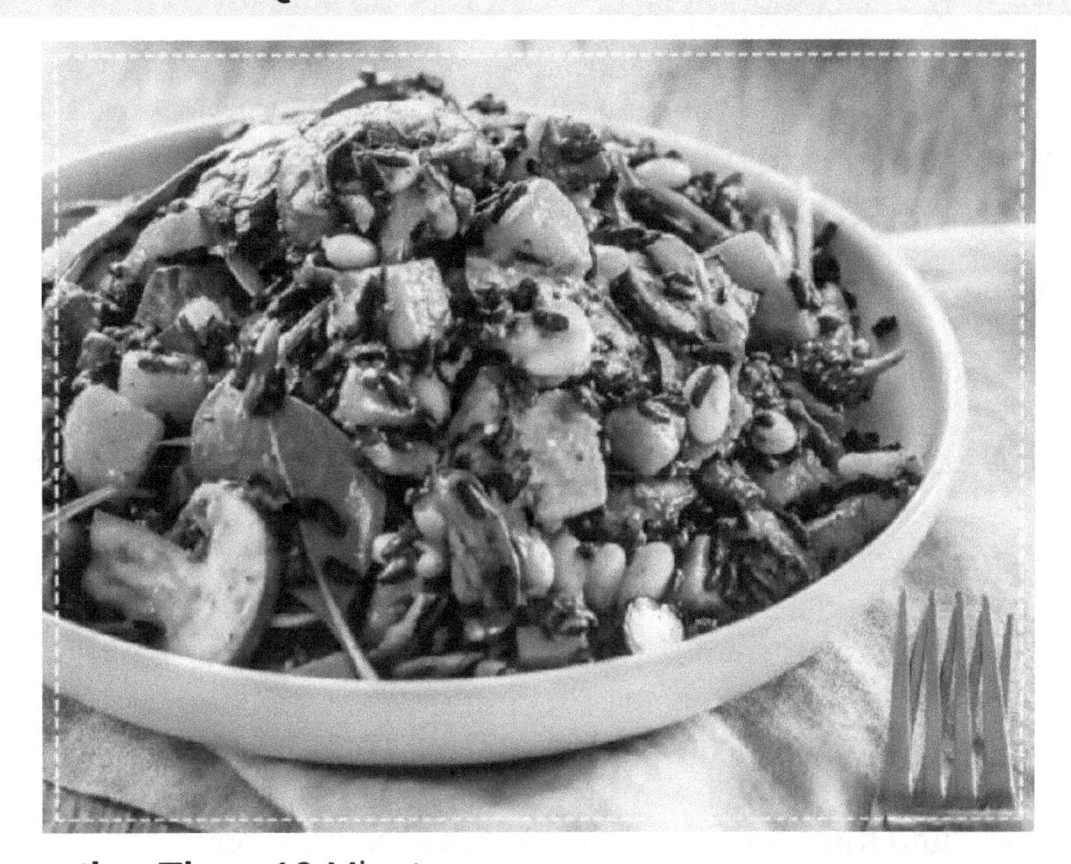

Preparation Time: 10 Minutes
Cooking Time: 25 Minutes
Skill: Beginner
Serving Size: 8

INGREDIENTS:

For the salad:

- 10 oz. Mushrooms, sliced
- 2 cups Black Rice, dried
- 1 lb. Butternut Squash, chopped
- 2 tbsp. Olive Oil
- ¼ cup Cranberries, dried
- ¼ cup Pumpkin Seeds
- 6 oz. Spinach, fresh & chopped
- 15 oz. White Beans, cooked
- Black Pepper, as needed

For the peanut dressing:

- ¼ cup Almond Milk
- 1 cup Coconut Cream
- 1/3 cup Rice Vinegar
- ¼ cup Extra Virgin Olive Oil
- 2 tbsp. Curry Paste

COOKING INSTRUCTION:

- Preheat the oven to 400 °F.
- After that, put the squash, pepper, and olive oil in a
- baking pan. Toss them once or twice so that the oil and pepper coat the squash well.
- Now, roast the squash for 10 to 15 minutes or until cooked. Set it aside.
- In the meantime, cook the black rice until al dente. Keep it
- aside. Next, mix all the ingredients needed to make the peanut dressing in another bowl until smooth.
- Finally, combine the roasted squash, cooked rice, and the remaining ingredients in a large bowl.
- Spoon the dressing over the ingredients and serve immediately.

Tip: If possible, use red curry paste.

NUTRITIONAL INFORMATION PER SERVING:

- Calories: 618 Kcal
- Protein: 22.2g
- Carbohydrates: 85.1g
- Fat: 24.1g

WHITE BEAN & AVOCADO SALAD

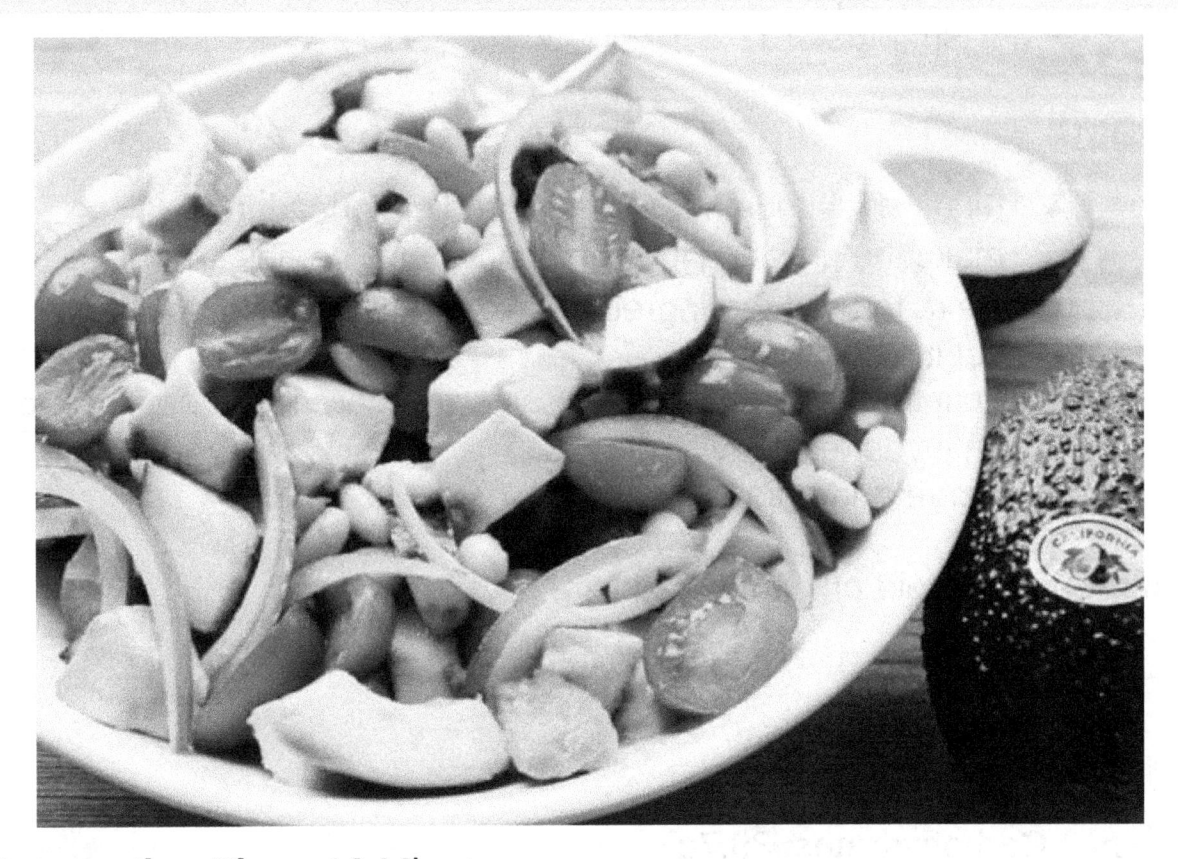

Preparation Time: 10 Minutes
Cooking Time: 10 Minutes
Skill: Beginner
Serving Size: 2 to 4

INGREDIENTS:

- 14 oz. White Beans
- 1 Avocado, chopped
- 1 Roma Tomato, chopped
- ¼ of 1 Sweet Onion, chopped

For the vinaigrette:

- 1 ½ tbsp. Olive Oil
-
- ¼ cup Lemon Juice
- ½ tsp. Garlic, finely chopped

- Fresh Basil, as needed, for garnish
- Salt & Pepper, to taste
- 1 tsp. Mustard

COOKING INSTRUCTIONS:

- First, whisk together all the ingredients needed to make the dressing in a small bowl until combined well.
- Next, toss all the ingredients in a large mixing bowl and set it aside.
- Pour the vinaigrette over the salad and place it in the refrigerator until you're ready to serve.
- Serve and enjoy.

Tip: You can avoid onion if you desire.

NUTRITIONAL INFORMATION PER SERVING:

- Calories: 452Kcal
- Protein: 13.3g
- Carbohydrates: 39.7g
- Fat: 28.7g

SPRING WATERMELON RADISH SALAD

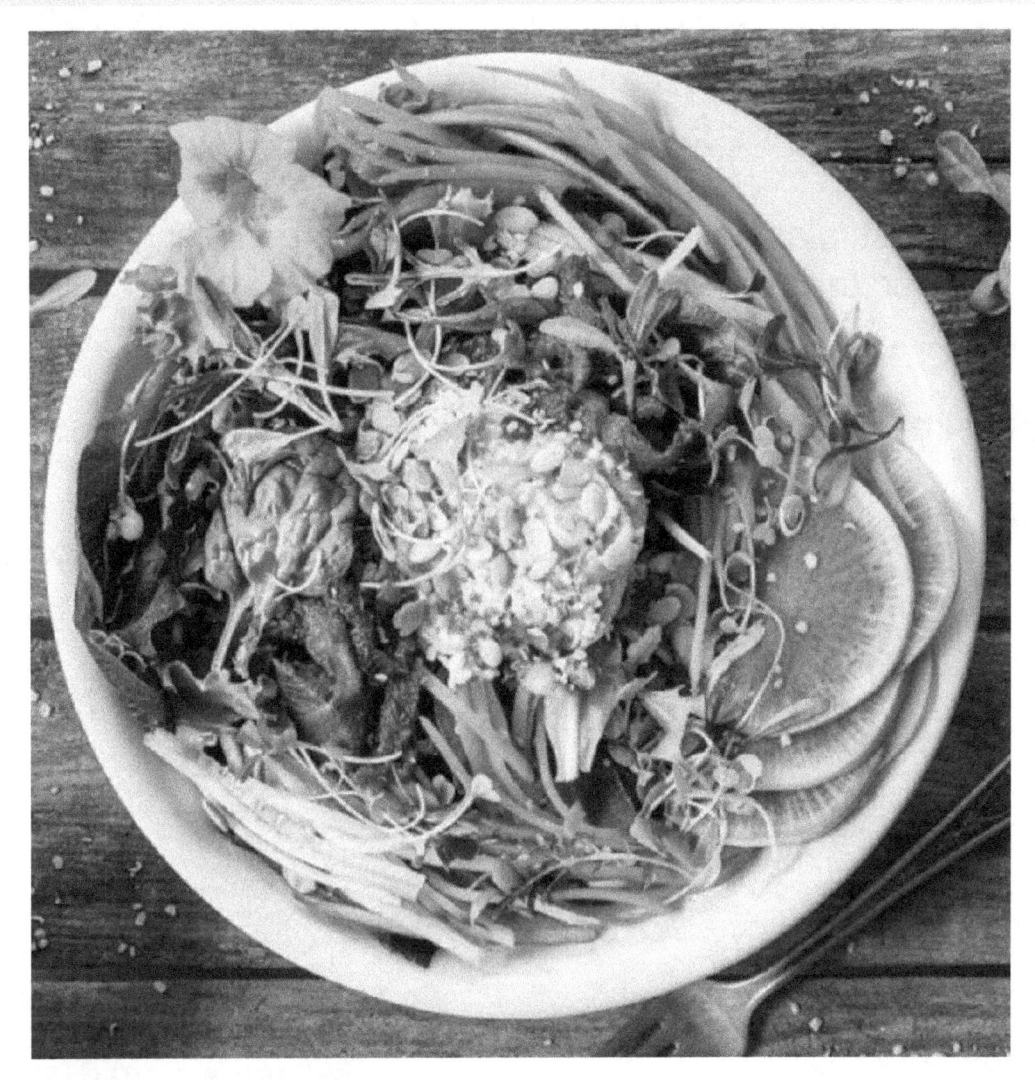

Preparation Time: 10 Minutes
Cooking Time: 10 Minutes
Skill: Beginner
Serving Size: 1

INGREDIENTS:

For the salad:

- 1 Watermelon Radish, sliced thinly
- ½ cup Hummus
- 2 tbsp. Pepitas
- 2 cups Spring Mix Greens

- 1 tbsp. Hemp Hearts
- ¼ cup Sun-dried Tomatoes
- 2 Carrots, medium & julienned
- 1/3 English Cucumber, cubed

COOKING INSTRUCTION:

- First, place all the ingredients in a large mixing bowl and toss them well.
- Serve immediately.

Tip: If desired, you can use microgreens also.

NUTRITIONAL INFORMATION PER SERVING:

- Calories: 629 Kcal
- Protein: 31g
- Carbohydrates: 63g
- Fat: 33g

SAVORY PROTEIN SNACKS

CHOC CHICKPEA COOKIES

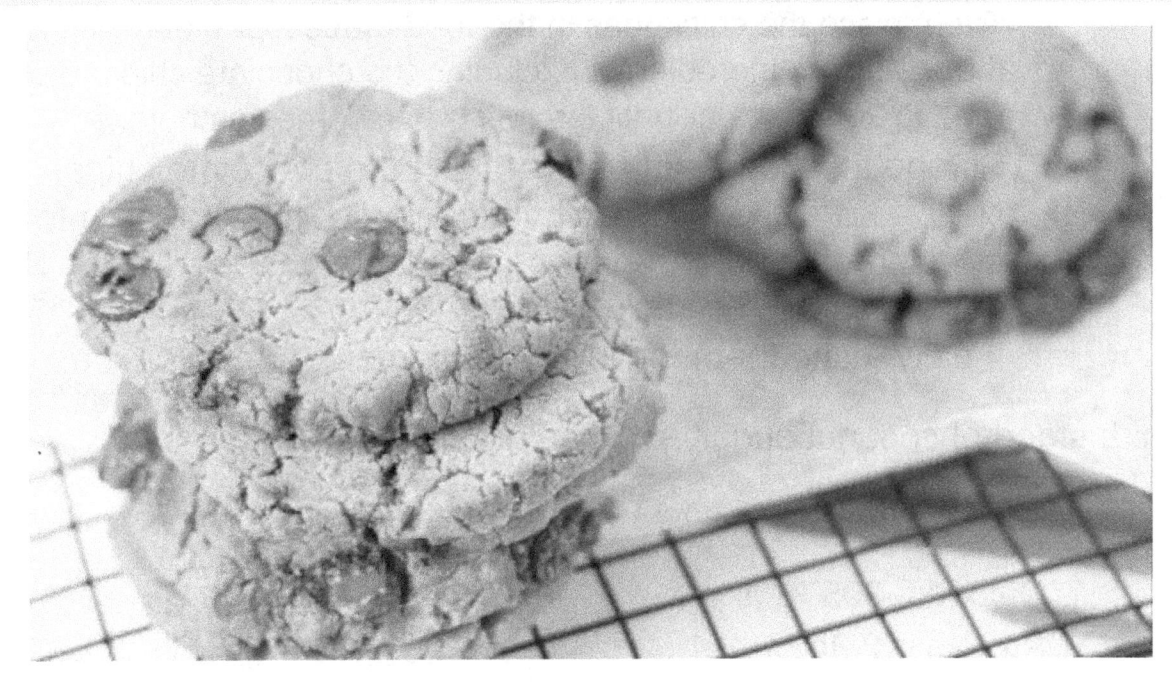

Preparation Time: 10 Minutes
Cooking Time: 1 Hour 30 Minutes
Skill: Beginner
Serving Size: 10

INGREDIENTS:

- ¼ tsp. Cinnamon
- 15 oz. Chickpeas, washed & drained
- 1/3 cup Chocolate Chips
- ½ cup Peanut Butter, creamy
- ¼ tsp. Salt
- 1/3 cup Coconut Sugar
- 1 Banana, small & overripe
- 1 tsp. Baking Powder
- 2 tsp. Vanilla Extract
- 2 tbsp. Flaxseed, grounded

COOKING INSTRUCTION:

- First, preheat the oven to 350 °F.
- After that, clean the chickpeas thoroughly and drain away all the excess water.
- Then, place the chickpeas in the food processor along with all the remaining ingredients, excluding the chocolate chips. Blend
- for 1 to 2 minutes or until the mixture becomes smooth.
- Scrape the sides and gently fold in the chocolate chips.
- Now, using your oiled hands, place the batter into a greased parchment paper-lined baking sheet. Tip: The mixture should be sticky.
- Finally, bake them for 11 to 12 minutes or until cooked.

Tip: Instead of coconut sugar, you can use any sugar.

NUTRITIONAL INFORMATION PER SERVING:

- Calories: 305 Kcal
- Protein: 12.3g
- Carbohydrates: 41.6g
- Fat: 11.2g

CHERRY VANILLA PROTEIN BARS

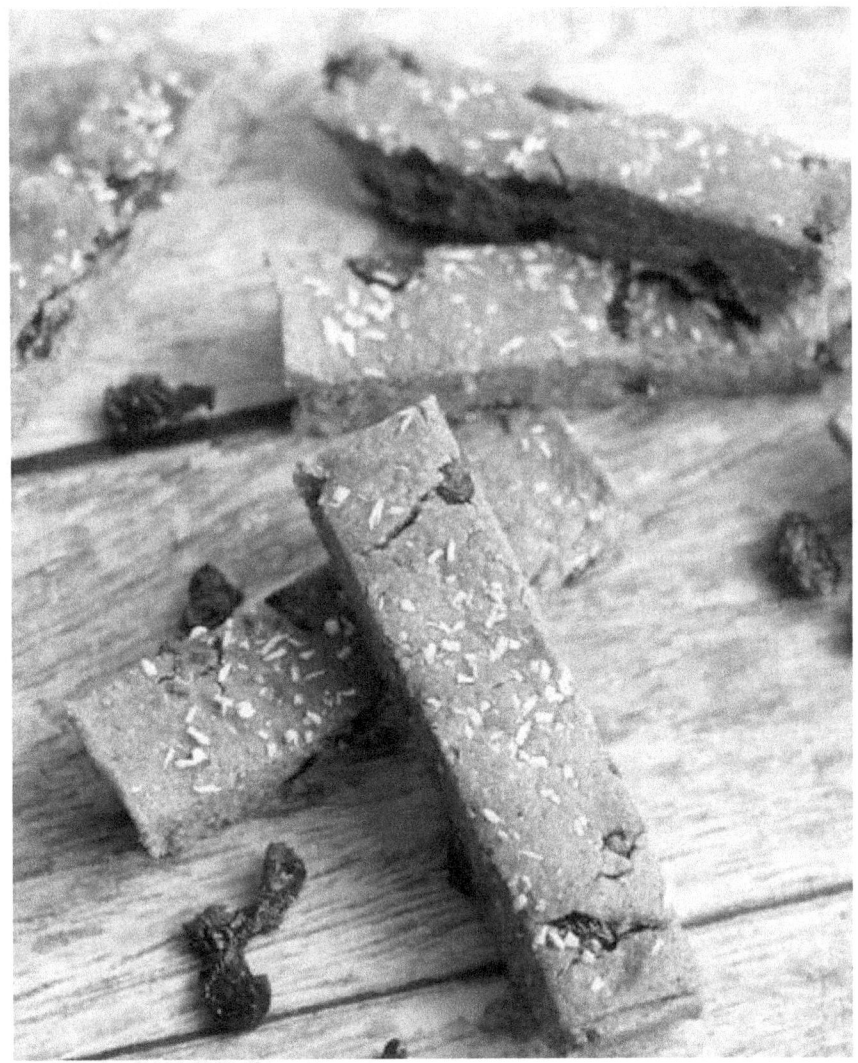

Preparation Time: 10 Minutes
Cooking Time: 10 Minutes
Skill: Beginner
Serving Size: 11 Bars

INGREDIENTS:

- 1 tbsp. Vanilla Extract
- 1 cup Oats
- 1/3 cup Cranberries, dried
- 1/3 cup Flaxseed, grounded
- ½ cup Almond Butter

- 1/3 cup Shredded Coconut, unsweetened
- ¼ cup Maple Syrup, pure
- 3 scoop Vegan Protein Powder

COOKING INSTRUCTION:

- To start with, combine the oats, protein powder, flaxseed, and coconut in a high-speed blender. Process for 3 minutes or until finely ground.
- After that, place the oat mixture into a large mixing bowl.
- Stir in the almond butter, vanilla, maple syrup, and almond milk.
- Mix well until combined.
- Now, gently fold in the cherries and give everything a good
- stir. Next, place the batter onto a greased parchment paper-lined baking sheet and press down slightly with your fingers until smooth and even.
- Finally, place in the freezer for a half-hour or until set.

Tip: Instead of dried cherries, you can also use dried cranberries.

NUTRITIONAL INFORMATION PER SERVING:

- Calories: 120 Kcal
- Protein: 7.2g
- Carbohydrates: 11.5g
- Fat: 4.6g

KALE PAPRIKA CHIPS

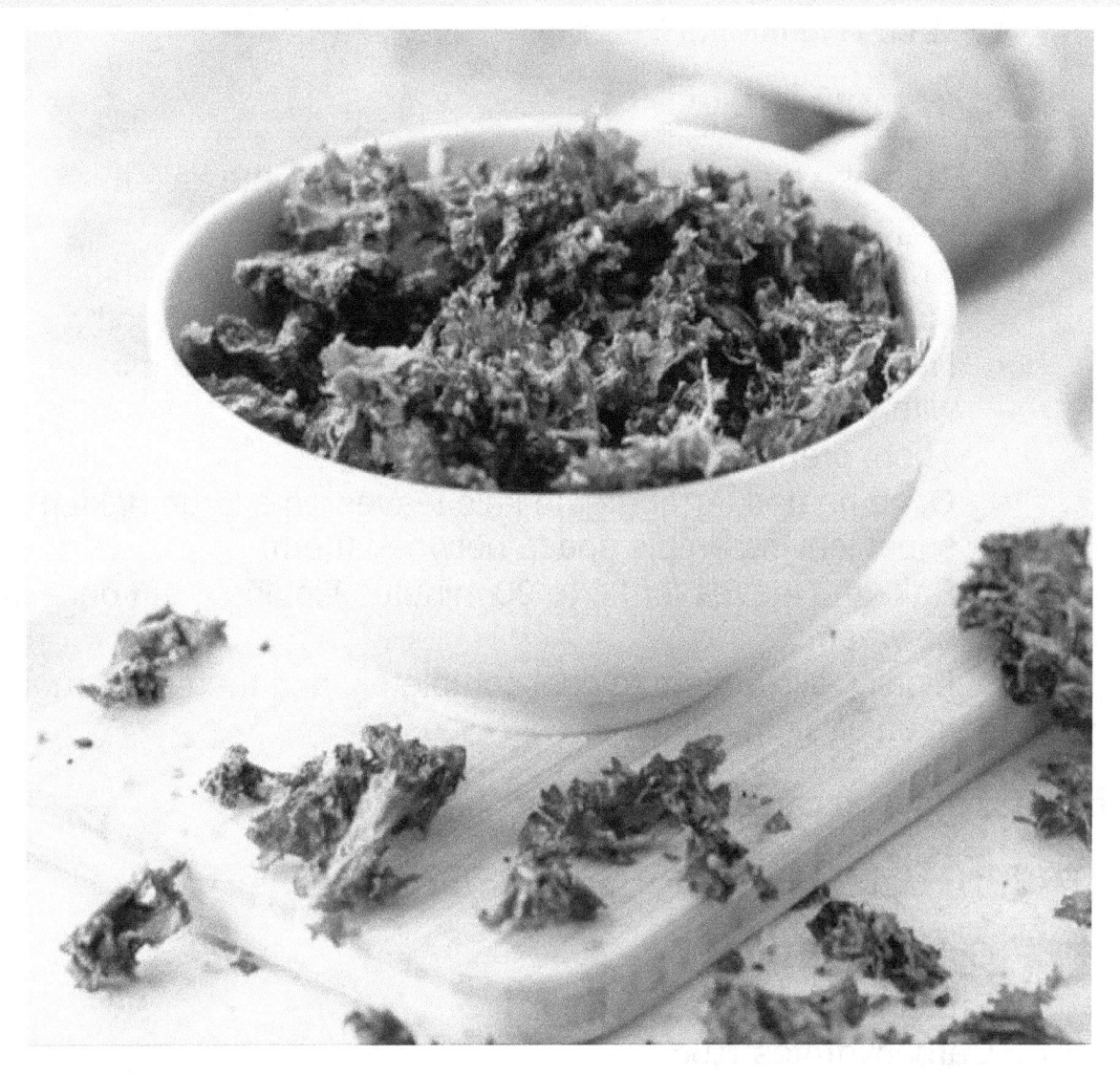

Preparation Time: 10 Minutes
Cooking Time: 1 Hour 30 Minutes
Skill: Beginner
Serving Size: 10

INGREDIENTS:

- ½ tsp. Smoked Paprika
- 2 bunches of Curly Kale
- 1 tsp. Garlic Powder
- ½ cup Nutritional Yeast

- 2 cups Cashew, soaked for 2 hours
- 1 tsp. Salt
- ½ cup Nutritional Yeast

COOKING INSTRUCTION:

- To make these tasty, healthy chips place the kale in a large mixing bowl.
- Now, combine all the remaining ingredients in the high-speed blender and blend for 1 minute or until smooth.
- Next, pour this dressing over the kale chips and mix well with your hands.
- Then, preheat your oven to 225 ° F or 107 °C.
- Once heated, arrange the kale leaves on a large baking sheet leaving ample space between them.
- Bake the leaves for 80 to 90 minutes flipping them once in between.
- Finally, allow them to cool completely and then store them in an air-tight container.

Tip: If desired, you can add more cayenne powder.

NUTRITIONAL INFORMATION PER SERVING:

- Calories: 191Kcal
- Protein: 9g
- Carbohydrates: 16g
- Fat: 12g

VANILLA ALMONDS HEMP PROTEIN BARS

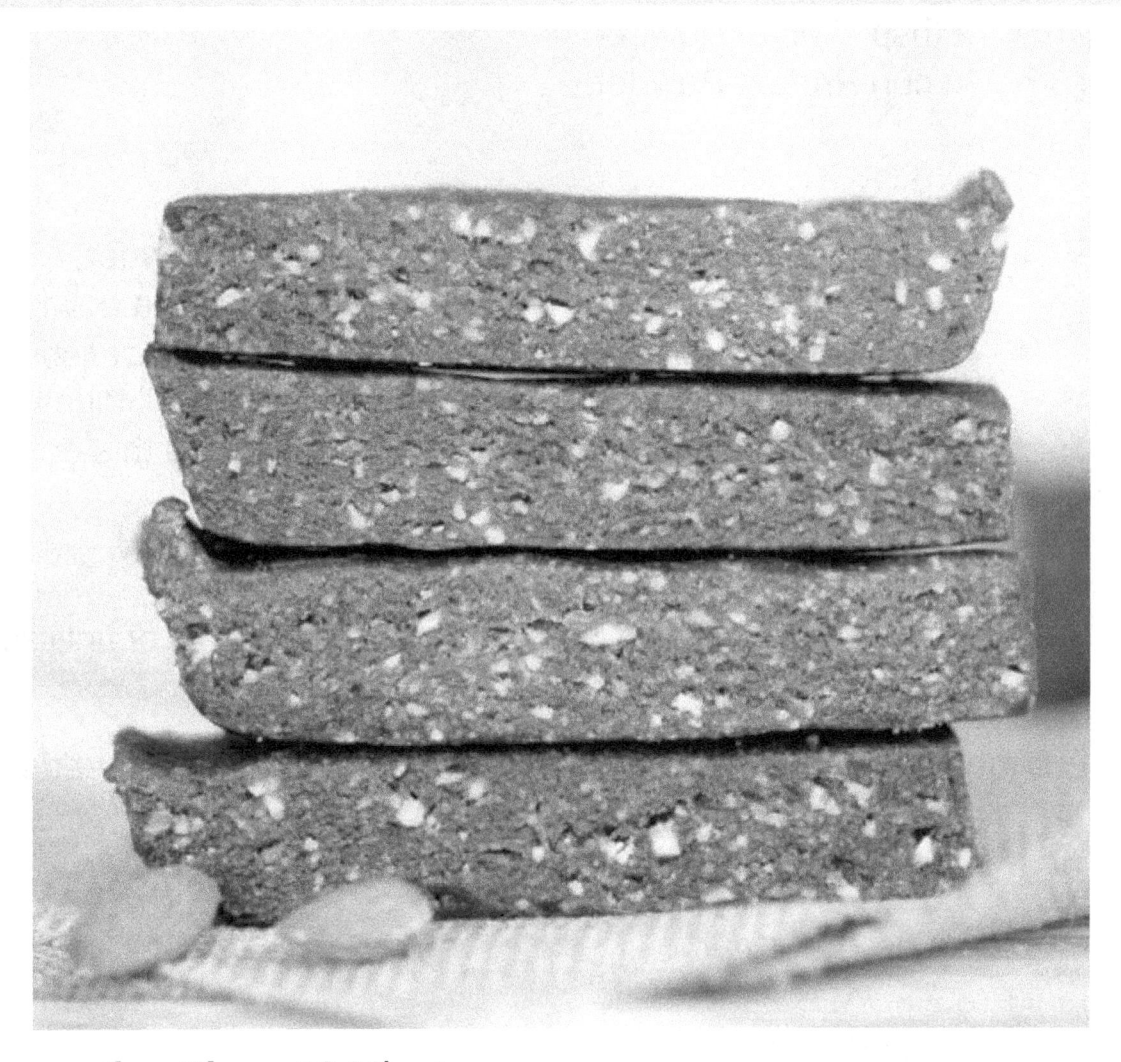

Preparation Time: 10 Minutes
Cooking Time: 30 Minutes
Skill: Beginner
Serving Size: 12 Bars

INGREDIENTS:

- 3 tbsp. Hemp Seeds
- 1 cup raw Almonds
- 1/3 cup Raw Seeds, mixed
- ½ tsp. Vanilla
- 2 tbsp. Water
- ½ cup Coconut, shredded & unsweetened

- 2 tbsp. Water
- 1 cup Medjool Dates
- 2 tbsp. Cacao Powder
- ¼ cup Protein Powder

COOKING INSTRUCTION:

- To begin with, place the mixed nuts, protein powder, water, shredded coconut, and hemp seeds into a bowl.
- Next, stir the dates, vanilla, and cacao into the processor. Blend for a minute or until everything is mixed well together.
- Now, add the reserved nut and seed mixture to this date mixture mix until everything is combined.
- Then, spread the mixture evenly over the greased parchment paper-lined baking sheet.
- Finally, place the mixture in the freezer for 2 hours or until set.
- Slice into squares.

Tip: For the raw seeds, you can use sunflower and pumpkin seeds.

NUTRITIONAL INFORMATION PER SERVING:

- Calories: 120 Kcal
- Protein: 7.2g
- Carbohydrates: 11.5g
- Fat: 4.6g

SPICY SQUASH SEEDS

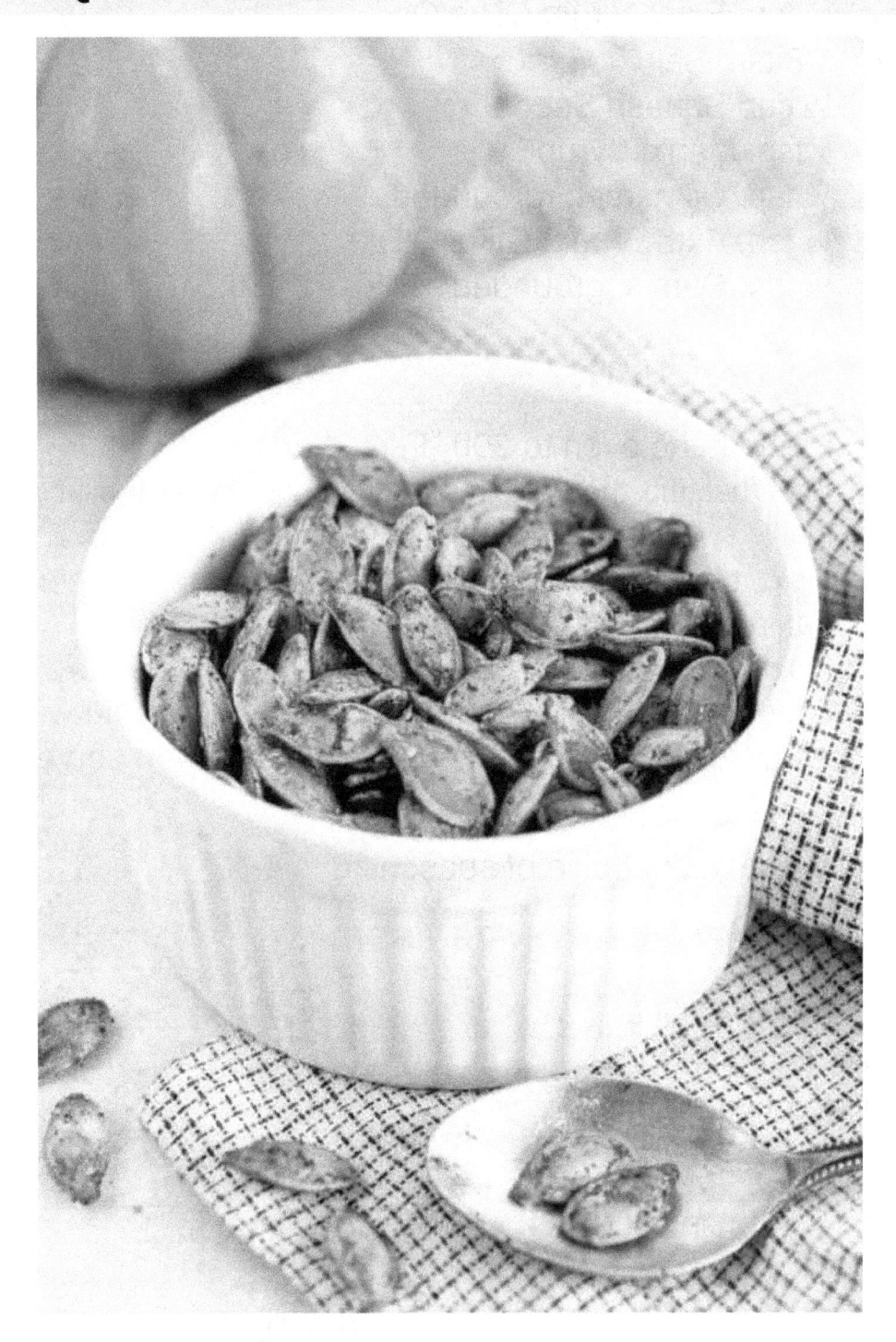

Preparation Time: 5 Minutes
Cooking Time: 50 Minutes
Skill: Beginner
Serving Size: 2

INGREDIENTS:

- ½ tsp. Extra Virgin Olive Oil
- 1/8 tsp. Salt
- ½ cup Squash Seeds
- 1 tsp. Maple Syrup
- ½ tsp. Cinnamon, grounded
- ½ tsp. Extra Virgin Olive Oil
- ½ tsp. Cumin, grounded

COOKING INSTRUCTIONS:

- Preheat the oven to 300 °F.
- After that, mix the squash seeds with cumin, olive oil, cinnamon, maple syrup, and salt in a large mixing bowl. Toss well.
- Next, transfer them to a greased parchment paper-lined baking sheet and spread it evenly.
- Now, bake them for 10 to 15 minutes or until they are crispy and golden colored. Stir them once in between.
- Allow the seeds to cool completely and then serve.

Tip: You can add your choice of seasoning to it.

NUTRITIONAL INFORMATION PER SERVING:

- Calories: 203cal
- Proteins: 10g
- Carbohydrates: 6g
- Fat: 17g

SOUPS

BASIC RECIPE FOR VEGETABLE BROTH

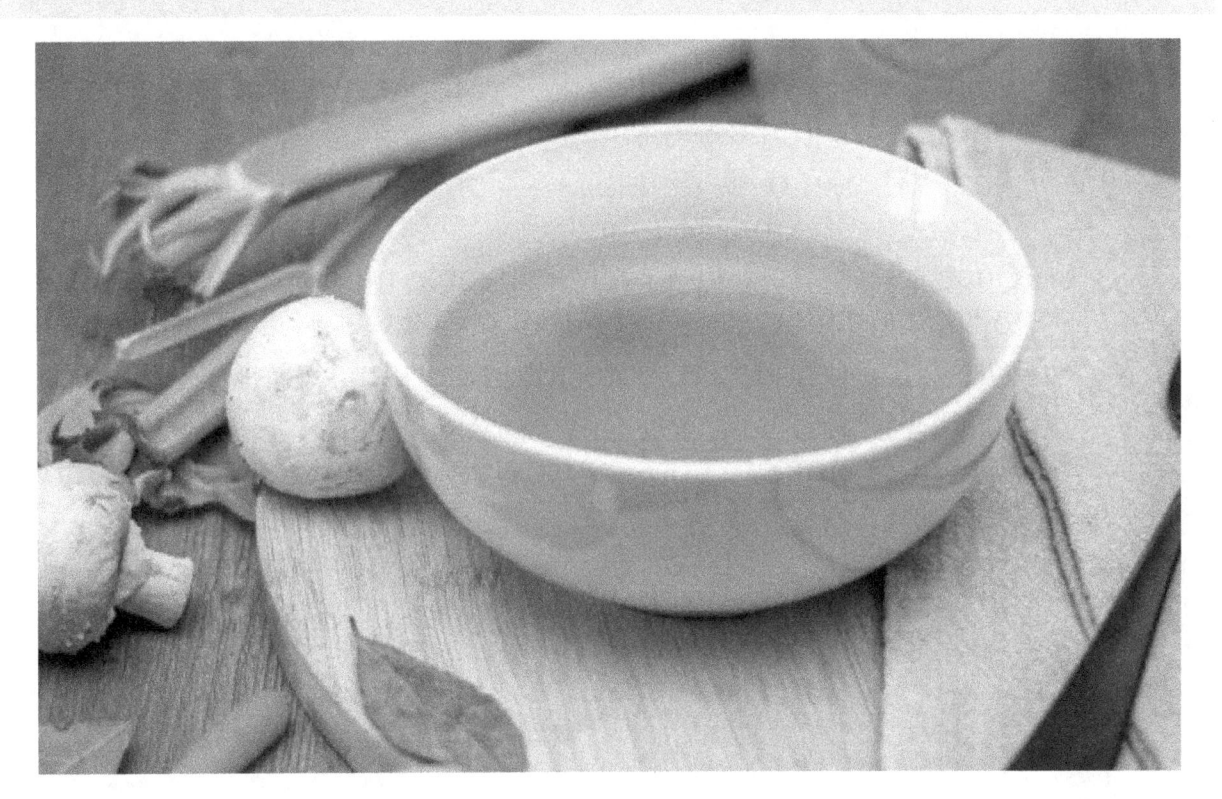

Preparation Time: 10 Minutes
Cooking Time: 60 Minutes
Skill: Beginner
Serving Size: Makes 2 Quarts

Ingredients:

- 8 cups Water
- 1 Carrot, chopped
- 1 Potato, medium & chopped
- 1 Onion, chopped
- 4 Garlic cloves, crushed
- 2 Celery Stalks, chopped
- Pinch of Salt
- Dash of Pepper
- 1 tbsp. Soy Sauce

- 3 Bay Leaves

COOKING INSTRUCTION:

- To make the vegetable broth, you need to place all of the ingredients in a deep saucepan.
- Heat the pan over a medium-high heat. Bring the vegetable mixture to a boil.
- Once it starts boiling, lower the heat to medium-low and allow it to simmer for at least an hour or so. Cover it with a lid.
- When the time is up, pass it through a filter and strain the vegetables, garlic, and bay leaves.
- Allow the stock to cool completely and store in an air-tight container.

Tip: If desired, you can even add mushrooms to it.

NUTRITIONAL INFORMATION PER SERVING:

- Calories: 4oKcal
- Protein: 1 g
- Carbohydrates: 9g
- Fat: 0g

CREAMY WHITE BEAN SOUP

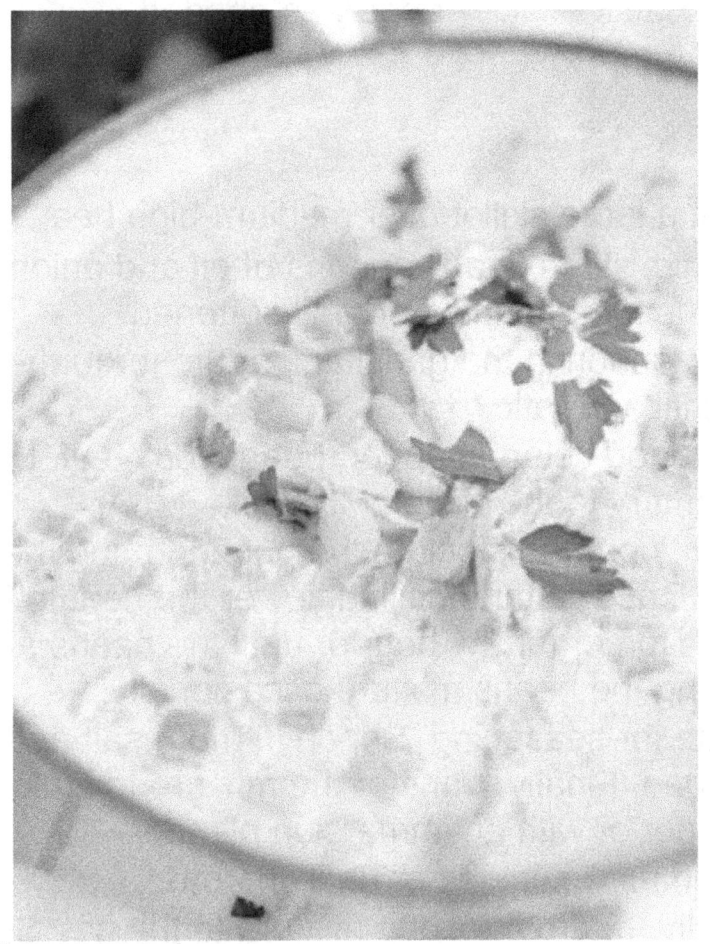

Preparation Time: 10 Minutes
Cooking Time: 80 Minutes
Skill: Beginner
Serving Size: 4

INGREDIENTS:

- 1 sprig of Parsley
- 4 tbsp. Olive Oil
- 1 Bay Leaf
- 1 cup Cannellini Beans, soaked for overnight & drained
- 1 Onion, large & chopped
- 1 Celery, large & chopped
- 2 Garlic Cloves, minced
- 1 tbsp. Lemon Juice

- 4 cups Vegetable Stock
- 1 sprig of Thyme
- Sea Salt & Black Pepper, as needed
- 1 sprig of Rosemary

COOKING INSTRUCTIONS:

- Heat a large skillet over medium-high heat.
- To this, stir in 2 tablespoons of oil and onion. Saute the onions for 4 minutes or until softened.
- Now, spoon in the garlic and sauté for further one minute or until aromatic.
- Next, add celery, pepper, beans, bay leaf, thyme, and rosemary to the skillet. Mix well.
- Then, pour the stock to the pot and bring the mixture to a
- boil. Once it starts boiling, lower the heat to low and allow it to simmer for 1½ hour or until the beans are soft while stirring the beans mixture occasionally.
- Taste for seasoning. Spoon in more salt and pepper if
- needed. Finally, transfer the mixture to a high-speed blender or with an immersion blender.
- Blend for 2 minutes or until smooth.
- Finally, return the soup mixture to the pot. Spoon the lemon juice and olive oil over it. Mix and serve it hot.

Tip: Garnish with rosemary if desired.

NUTRITIONAL INFORMATION PER SERVING:

- Calories: 316Kcal
- Proteins: 16g
- Carbohydrates: 53g
- Fat: 5.9g

SPICY SUN-DRIED TOMATO SOUP

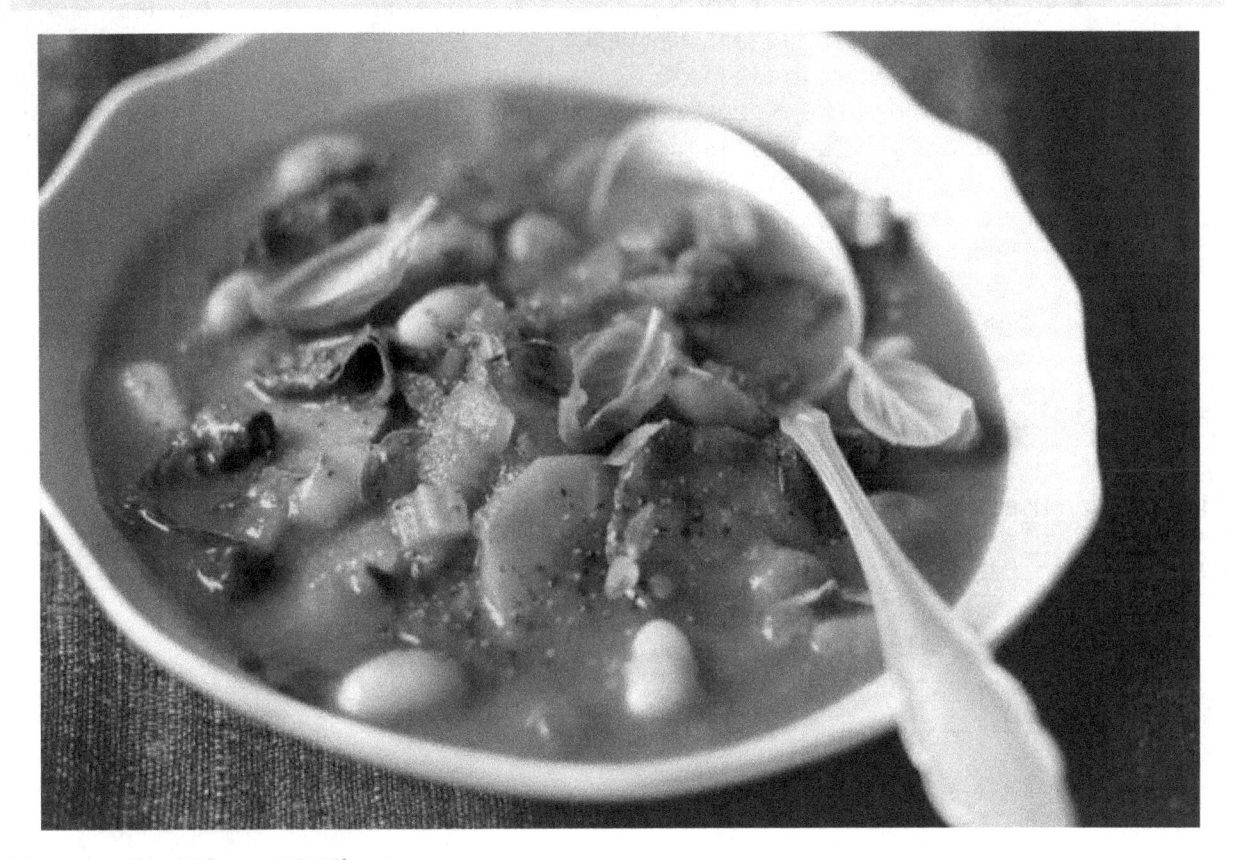

Preparation Time: 10 Minutes
Cooking Time: 35 Minutes
Skill: Beginner
Serving Size: 6

INGREDIENTS:

- 2-3 cloves of Garlic, minced
- 1 Carrot, medium and julienned
- 2 × 16 oz. Garbanzo Beans, divided
- 1 White Onion, small & chopped
- 2 cups Water
- 1 ½ tbsp. Olive Oil
- ½ cup Sun-dried Tomatoes in Oil
- 2 tsp. Rosemary, dried
- Pinch of Salt
- 1 Bay Leaf
- Dash of Pepper
- ½ tsp. Red Pepper Flakes
- 1 cup Pasta Shells

COOKING INSTRUCTIONS:

- First, you need to cook the pasta by following the instructions given in the packet.
- In the meantime, heat olive oil in a large skillet over medium-high heat.
- Once the oil becomes hot, stir in the red pepper flakes, onion, bay leaf, garlic, and rosemary to it. Mix well.
- Now, pour water to the mixture along with sun-dried tomatoes, garbanzo beans, and carrot. Keep 1 cup of beans aside.
- Next, bring the beans-veggie mixture to a boil and lower the heat to low.
- Cover the skillet with a lid. Allow it to simmer for 6 to 7 minutes. Set it aside for a few minutes.
- Then, transfer the beans mixture to a high-speed blender once slightly cooled.
- Blend for a minute or until it is finely pureed.
- Return the pureed mixture to the skillet over medium-low heat.
- Finally, add the cooked pasta and the reserved beans. Heat it through.
- Taste for seasoning. Add more salt and pepper if needed.
- Serve and enjoy.

Tip: You can use more water in the end, if the soup seems too thick.

NUTRITIONAL INFORMATION PER SERVING:

- Calories: 689Kcal
- Proteins: 38g
- Carbohydrates: 122g
- Fat: 7g

CREAMY BLACK BEAN SOUP

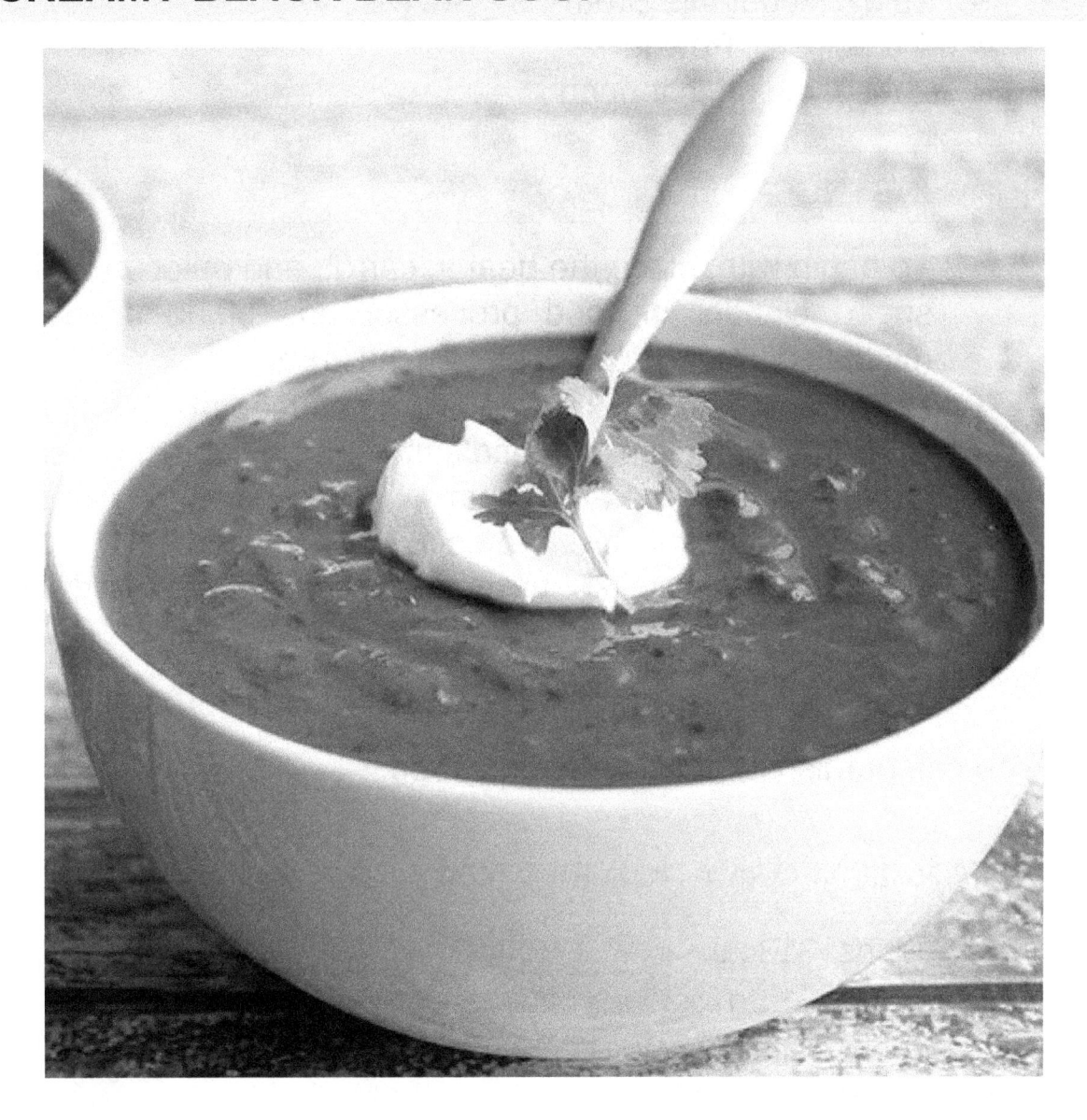

Preparation Time: 10 Minutes
Cooking Time: 15 Minutes
Skill: Beginner
Serving Size: 4

INGREDIENTS:

- 30 oz. Black Beans, cooked
- 1 Carrot, grated

- ½ cup Salsa
- 16 oz. Vegetable Broth
- 1 tbsp. Chili Powder
- 2 tbsp. Onion, chopped

COOKING INSTRUCTIONS:

- To begin with, place the beans, carrot, and onion in a high-speed blender or food processor and blend it for two minutes or until you get a smooth mixture.
- Now, transfer this mixture to a large saucepan.
- Heat it over medium heat and then to this, spoon in the salsa along with the vegetable broth.
- Next, bring the mixture to a boil.
- Once it starts boiling, take the pan away from the heat. Add chili powder.
- Serve it hot.

Tip: You can garnish it with cilantro if desired.

NUTRITIONAL INFORMATION PER SERVING:

- Calories: 313cal
- Proteins: 21.9g
- Carbohydrates: 53.9g
- Fat: 2.2g

FARRO LENTIL SOUP

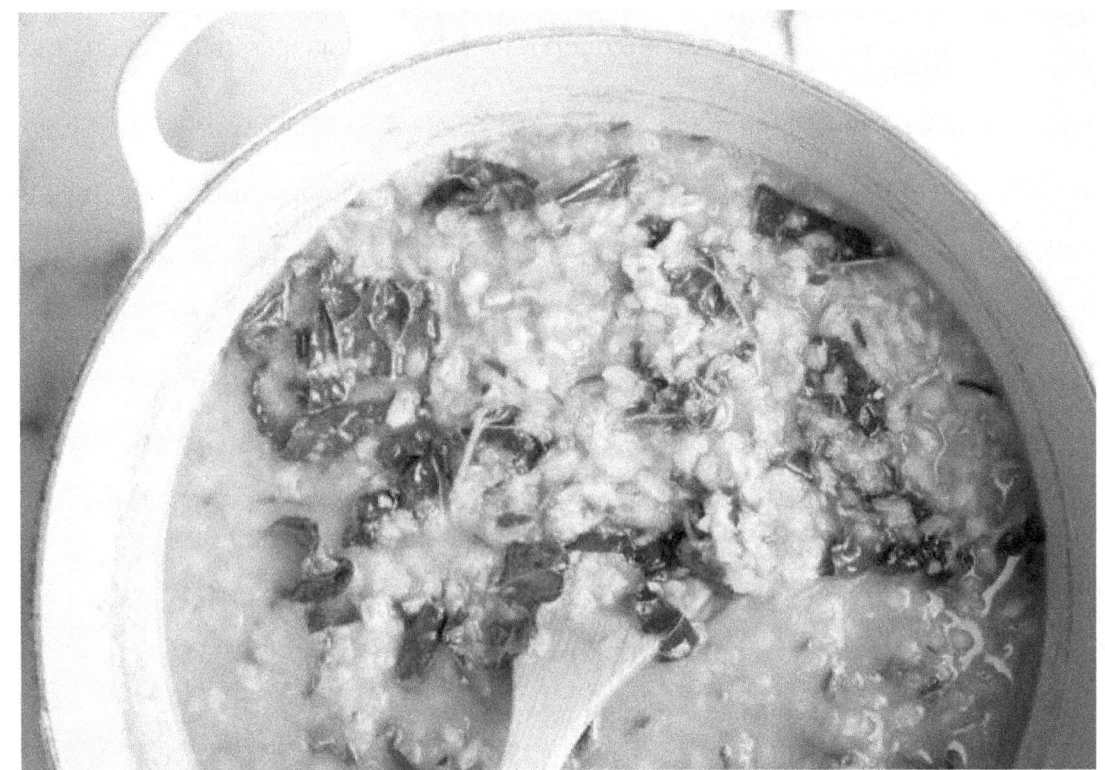

Preparation Time: 10 Minutes
Cooking Time: 30 Minutes
Skill: Beginner
Serving Size: 4

INGREDIENTS:

- 1 cup Kale, chopped
- ½ cup Farro, quick-cook
- 1½ tsp. Turmeric Powder
- 1 Onion, small & grated
- 2 tbsp. Olive Oil
- ½ cup Red Lentils
- 1 Zucchini, small and grated
- 5 cups Vegetable Broth
- 1½ tsp. Salt
- ½ tsp. Cumin
- ¼ tsp. Pepper
- 1 cup Carrot, grated

For the breadcrumbs:

- 1 Garlic clove
- 6 French Baguette slices
- 1 tsp. Olive Oil

- Salt, as needed

COOKING INSTRUCTIONS:

- Heat a large skillet over medium-high heat. To this, stir in the onion, zucchini, and carrot.
- After that, sauté the veggies for 2 to 3 minutes and then spoon in turmeric, pepper, cumin, and salt to the skillet.
- Once the mixture becomes aromatic, pour the broth to the veggie mixture.
- Now, bring the mixture to a boil. When it starts boiling, stir in the farro and
- lentils. Lower the heat. Allow the veggie mixture to simmer for 20 minutes or until the farro and lentils are cooked.
- In the meantime, for the breadcrumbs, place the bread slices and garlic in the food processor.
- Pulse them until you get small crumbs.
- Next, transfer the bread crumbs to a large baking sheet. Drizzle a bit of olive oil and salt over it. Toss well.
- Bake for 8 minutes or until the bread crumbs are golden brown.
- Finally, add the kale to the soup and cook until wilted.
- Serve it hot and top it with the toasted breadcrumbs.

Tip: Instead of kale, you can use any greens.

NUTRITIONAL INFORMATION PER SERVING:

- Calories: 428cal
- Proteins: 20.9g
- Carbohydrates: 59.7g
- Fat: 12.1g

GREEK LENTIL SOUP

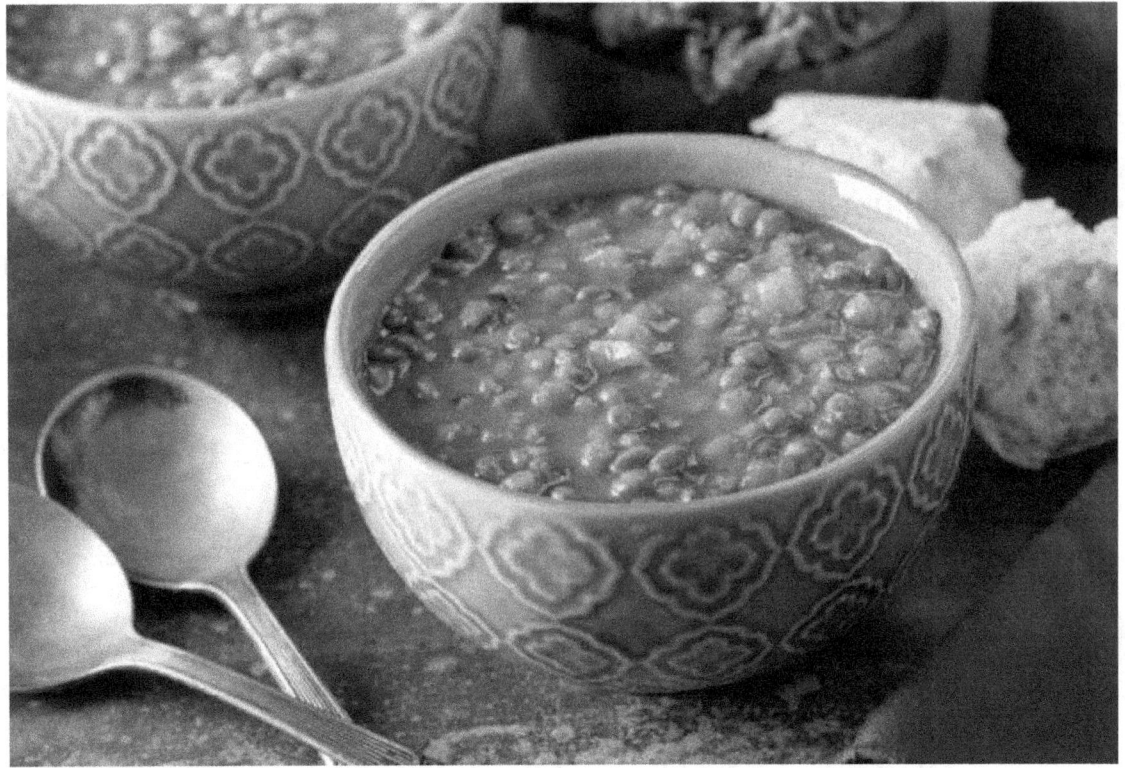

Preparation Time: 5 Minutes
Cooking Time: 30 Minutes
Skill: Beginner
Serving Size: 4

INGREDIENTS:

- 1 cup Carrot, diced
- 1 tsp. Salt
- 1 cup Lentils, dry
- 4 Lemon Wedges
- 1 tbsp. Olive Oil
- 2 Bay Leaves
- 1 tbsp. Red Wine Vinegar
- ½ cup Celery, diced
- 1 tsp. Black Pepper, grounded
- 1 cup Yellow Onion, diced
- 2 tbsp. Tomato Paste
- 4 Garlic cloves, minced

- 4 cups Vegetable Broth
- 3 tsp. Oregano, dried
- 1 tsp. Rosemary, grounded

COOKING INSTRUCTIONS:

- For making this delicious soup, boil a pot of water over medium-high heat.
- To this, stir in the lentils and cook for 4 to 5 minutes or until they are half cooked. Drain well.
- Heat olive oil in a large skillet, and once it becomes hot, add the celery, garlic, and onion.
- Saute them for 4 minutes or until they are translucent and fragrant.
- Now, pour the broth, rosemary, cooked lentils, oregano, and bay leaves.
- Bring the lentil mixture to a boil and lower the heat to
- simmer. Simmer the soup for 18 to 20 minutes or until the veggies are cooked and tender.
- In the meantime, discard the bay leaves and spoon in the tomato paste. Simmer for another five minutes.
- Finally, transfer the soup to the serving bowl and drizzle the red wine vinegar over it.
- Serve with lemon wedges and squeeze the juice if needed.

Tip: You can even serve it with toasted whole wheat pita bread.

NUTRITIONAL INFORMATION PER SERVING:

- Calories: 276Kcal
- Proteins: 15g
- Carbohydrates: 47g
- Fat: 5g

PUMPKIN & WHITE BEAN SOUP

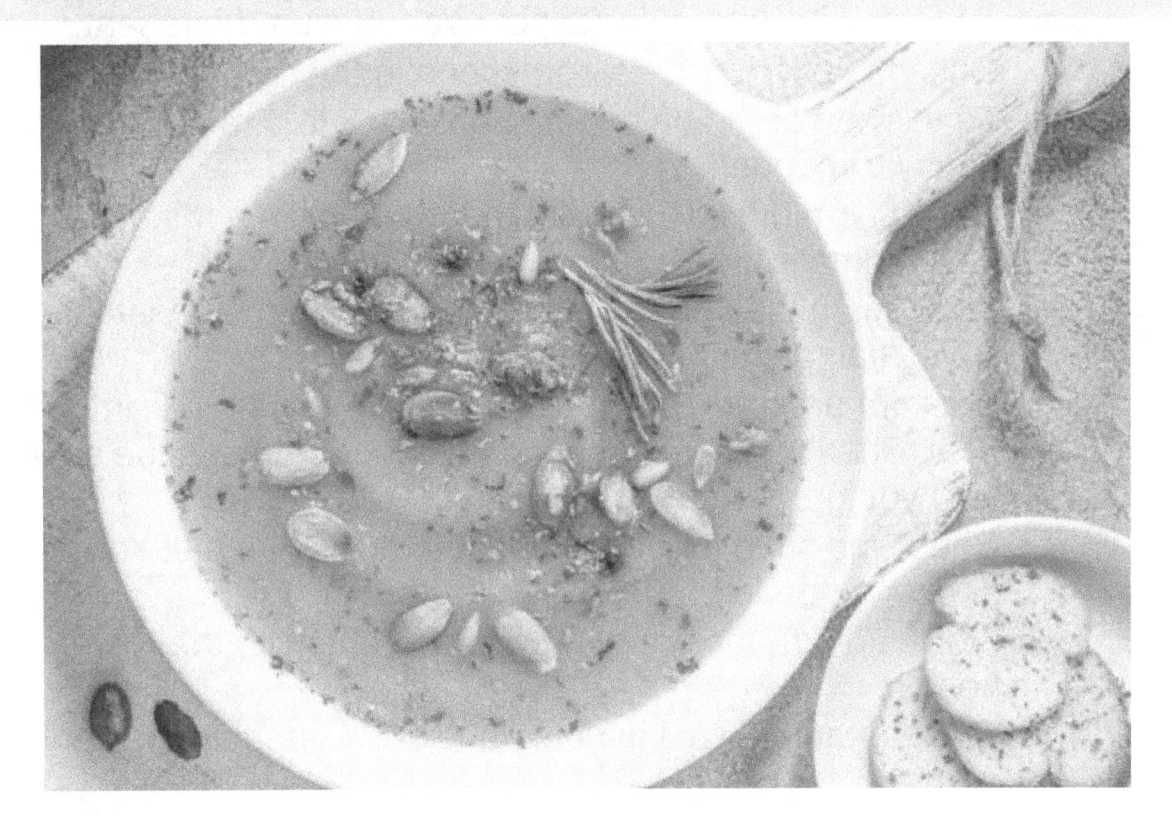

Preparation Time: 10 Minutes
Cooking Time: 20 Minutes
Skill: Beginner
Serving Size: 4

INGREDIENTS:

- 2 cups White Beans, cooked
- 1 tbsp. Olive Oil
- ½ cup Coconut Milk
- 2 cups Pumpkin Puree
- Salt & Pepper, as needed
- ½ of 1 Yellow Onion, diced
- 2 cups Water
- 2 Garlic cloves, minced
- ¼ cup Pumpkin Seeds, toasted
- 2 cups Vegetable Stock

COOKING INSTRUCTIONS:

- To start with, heat a large pot over medium-high heat.
- Once the pot becomes hot, spoon in the oil.
- To this, stir in the onion and cook for 3 to 4 minutes or until partially softened.
- Next, add the garlic and sauté for further one minute or until aromatic.
- Now, stir in the pumpkin puree along with the vegetable stock, half of the beans and water.
- Cook for another 13 minutes. Remove the soup from the
- heat. Then, with an immersion blender, process the soup until you get a smooth mixture.
- Check the soup for seasoning and add more salt and pepper if needed.
- Finally, return the soup to the pan along with the remaining beans.
- Cook for another 10 minutes and serve them in the serving bowls.
- Top with the pumpkin seeds and drizzle a bit of coconut milk over it.

Tip: To spice up the soup, you can add chilli powder to it.

NUTRITIONAL INFORMATION PER SERVING:

- Calories: 340cal
- Proteins: 14g
- Carbohydrates: 43g
- Fat: 14g

CREAMY BROCCOLI SOUP WITH CHICKPEAS

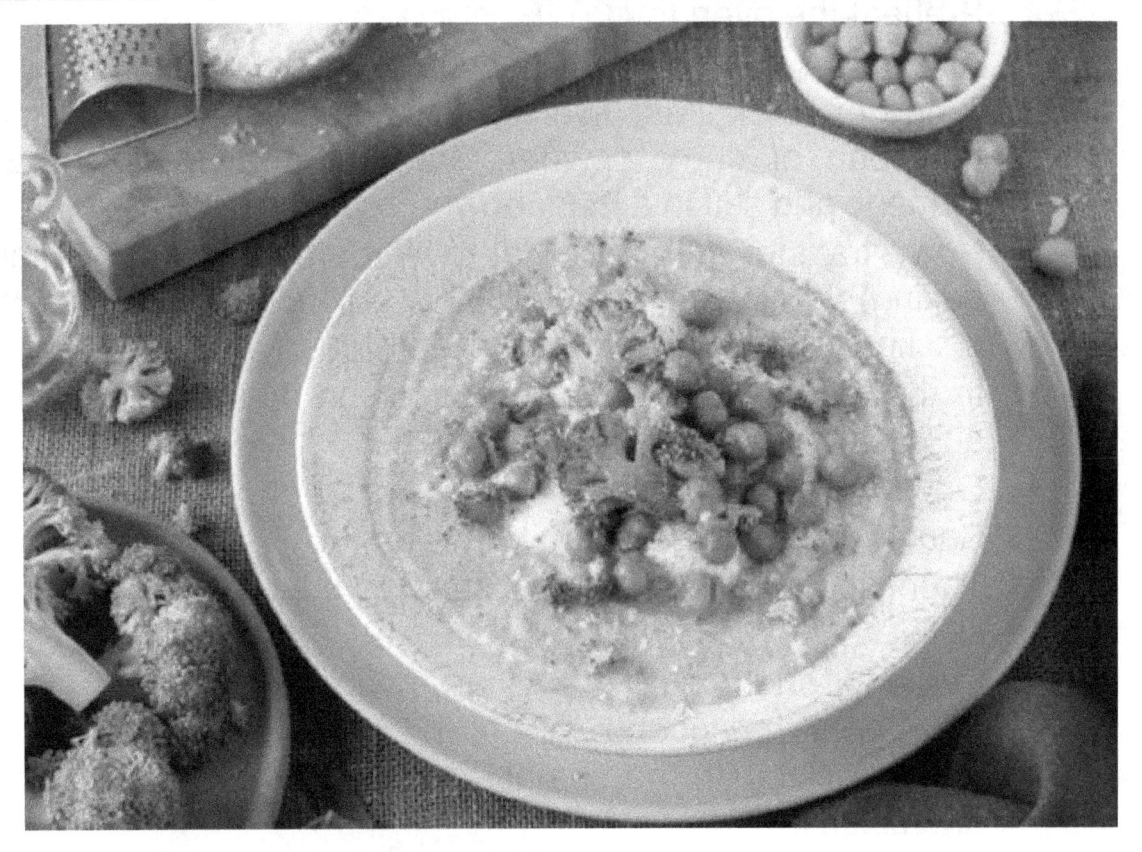

Preparation Time: 10 Minutes
Cooking Time: 15 Minutes
Skill: Beginner
Serving Size: 4
INGREDIENTS:

- 2 tbsp. Lemon Juice
- 1 Onion, large & chopped
- 1 lb. Broccoli, chopped
- 4 cups Vegetable Sock
- ¼ cup Coconut Oil
- 1 tsp. Turmeric
- 15 oz. Coconut Milk
- 2 tsp. Curry Powder
- 2 cloves of Garlic, minced
- Pinch of Sea Salt

COOKING INSTRUCTIONS:

- Preheat the oven to 400 °F.
- After that, take a cup of the broccoli and place it along with 1 cup of chickpeas, two tablespoons of coconut oil, one teaspoon of curry powder, and half teaspoon of each turmeric and salt in a large bowl. Toss well.
- Now, transfer this mixture to a parchment paper-lined baking sheet and bake for 10 to 15 minutes or until the chickpeas-broccoli becomes slightly crispy.
- In the meantime, spoon the remaining oil to a large skillet and heat it over medium-high heat.
- Once the oil becomes hot, stir in the onion.
- Sauté for 4 minutes or until translucent.
- Then, spoon in the turmeric, curry powder, and garlic to the skillet.
- Saute for one minute or until aromatic.
- Next, pour the coconut milk to the skillet. Scrap the bottom of the skillet with the spatula so that all the stuck portions are mixed in.
- Bring the chickpeas-broccoli mixture to a boil and lower the heat to medium-low.
- Allow the soup to simmer for 10 minutes or until the broccoli is tender.
- Take the skillet from the heat and spoon in the lemon
- juice. Finally, transfer the mixture to a food processor or by using an immersion blender; blend the soup until you get a
- smooth soup. Serve in serving bowls and top it with the crispy chickpeas and broccoli.

Tip: You can garnish it with cilantro if desired.

NUTRITIONAL INFORMATION PER SERVING:

- Calories: 600cal
- Proteins: 18g
- Carbohydrates: 48g
- Fat: 41g

CARROT & RED LENTIL SOUP

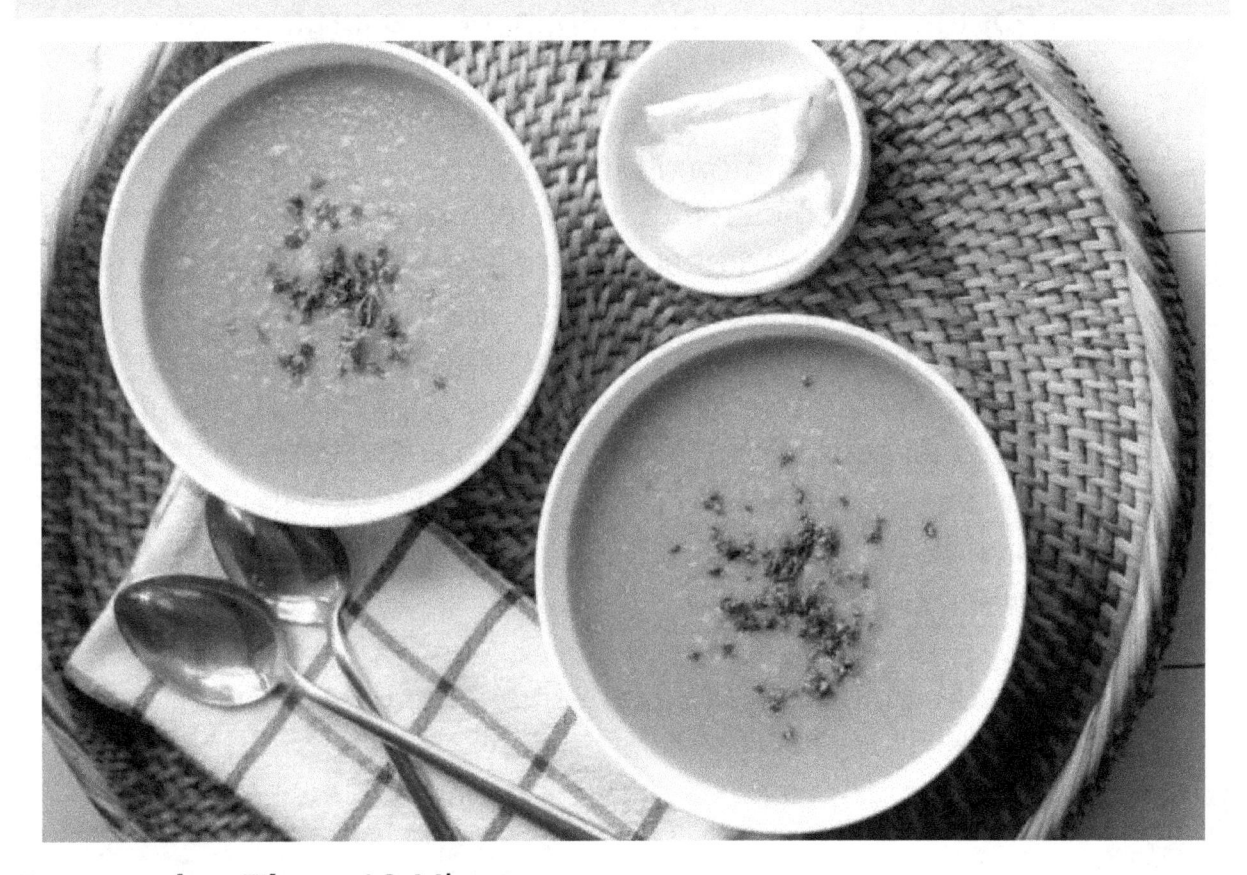

Preparation Time: 10 Minutes
Cooking Time: 25 Minutes
Skill: Beginner
Serving Size: 2

INGREDIENTS:

- 1 cup Red Lentils, dried
- 2 Carrot, chopped
- 1 tbsp. Olive Oil
- 5 cups Vegetable Broth
- 1 cup Tomato, pureed
- 1 Onion, chopped
- ½ tsp. Cumin, grounded
- 1 Garlic clove, grated

COOKING INSTRUCTIONS:

- For making this delicious soup, heat a large pot over medium heat.
- Once the oil becomes hot, spoon in the oil.
- To this, stir in the onion, carrot, and garlic.
- Sauté the onion-carrot for 2 minutes and then add the lentils to it.
- Continue cooking until the lentils are coated with the oil.
- Next, spoon in the tomato and cumin to the pot.
- Bring the veggie-tomato mixture to boil and allow it to simmer.
- Lower the heat to low and simmer for 18 to 20 minutes.
- Taste for seasoning. Spoon in more salt and pepper if required.
- Finally, blend it in a high-speed blender or with an immersion blender for 2 to 3 minutes.
- Serve hot.

Tip: You can add lemon juice to it for enhancing the flavor.

NUTRITIONAL INFORMATION PER SERVING:

- Calories: 534cal
- Proteins: 28g
- Carbohydrates: 79g
- Fat: 12g

LUNCH & DINNER

RED CABBAGE TACOS

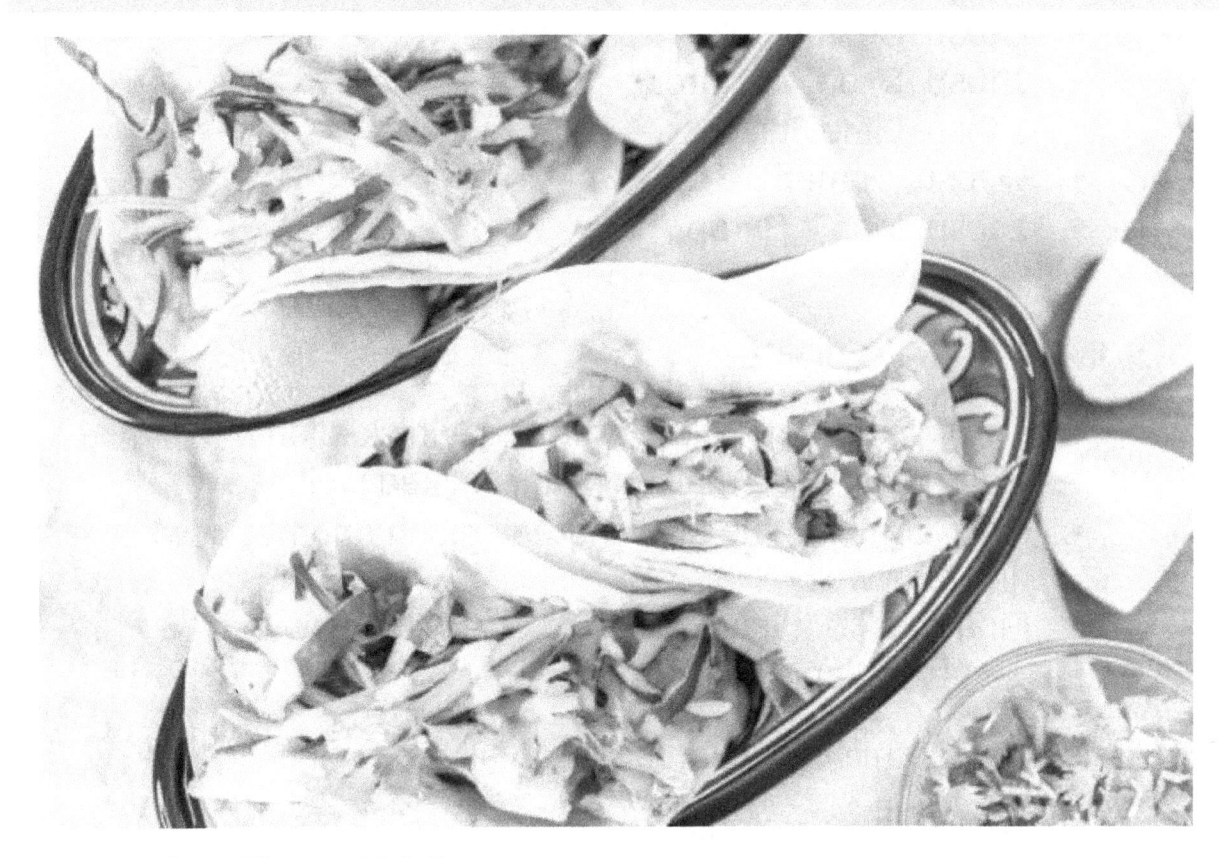

Preparation Time: 10 Minutes
Cooking Time: 30 Minutes
Skill: Beginner
Serving Size: 4

INGREDIENTS:

- 6 Taco Shells

For the slaw:

- 1 cup Red Cabbage, shredded
- 1 cup Green Cabbage, shredded
- 3 Scallions, chopped
- 1 cup Carrots, sliced

For the dressing:

- 1 tbsp. Sriracha
- ¼ cup Apple Cider Vinegar
- ¼ tsp. Salt
- 2 tbsp. Sesame Oil
- 1 tbsp. Dijon Mustard
- 1 tbsp. Lime Juice
- ½ tbsp. Tamari
- 1 tbsp. Maple Syrup
- ¼ tsp. Salt

COOKING INSTRUCTIONS:

- To start with, make the dressing, whisk all the ingredients in a small bowl until mixed well.
- Next, combine the slaw ingredients in another bowl and toss well.
- Finally, take a taco shell and place the slaw in it.
- Serve and enjoy.

Tip: Instead of soy milk, you can also use almond milk.

NUTRITIONAL INFORMATION PER SERVING:

- Calories: 216Kcal
- Protein: 10g
- Carbohydrates: 15g
- Fat: 13g

SPAGHETTI SQUASH WITH TEMPEH

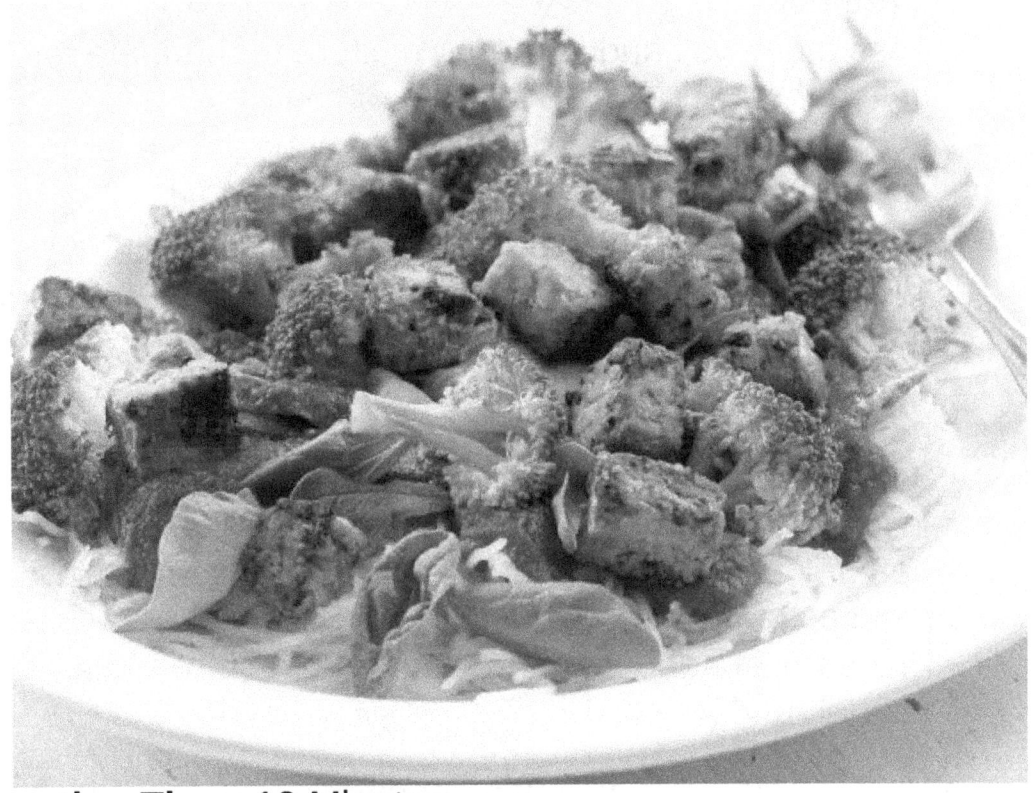

Preparation Time: 10 Minutes
Cooking Time: 45 Minutes
Skill: Beginner
Serving Size: 4

INGREDIENTS:

- 2 tbsp. Tamari
- 1 tbsp. Canola Oil
- 12 oz. Tempeh, cubed
- 25 oz. Pasta Sauce
- ¼ cup Mirin
- 2 ½ lb. Squash, halved lengthwise & seeded
- 1 cup Baby Spinach
- 2 cloves of Garlic, finely chopped
- 2 cups Broccoli Florets

COOKING INSTRUCTIONS:

- Preheat the oven to 375 ° F.
- After that, combine garlic, tempeh, and mirin in a medium-sized bowl.
- Toss them well and allow the mixture to marinate for half an hour.
- In the meantime, place the halved squash in a large baking sheet with the cut sides down.
- Next, bake them for 35 to 40 minutes or until tender.
- Once cooked, allow it to cool and spoon the insides with a fork to get our noodles.
- Then, heat oil in a large-sized saucepan over medium
- heat. Then, add the tempeh into the pan and cook for 8 minutes or until they are tender.
- In the meantime, place the pasta sauce over medium
- heat. Finally, stir in the broccoli and cook for further 5 minutes or until softened.
- Place the spaghetti on the plate and top it with the tempeh and broccoli.

Tip: Instead of sirin, you can also use honey.

NUTRITIONAL INFORMATION PER SERVING:

- Calories: 430Kcal
- Protein: 22g
- Carbohydrates: 50g
- Fat: 17g

VEGAN CHILI CARNE

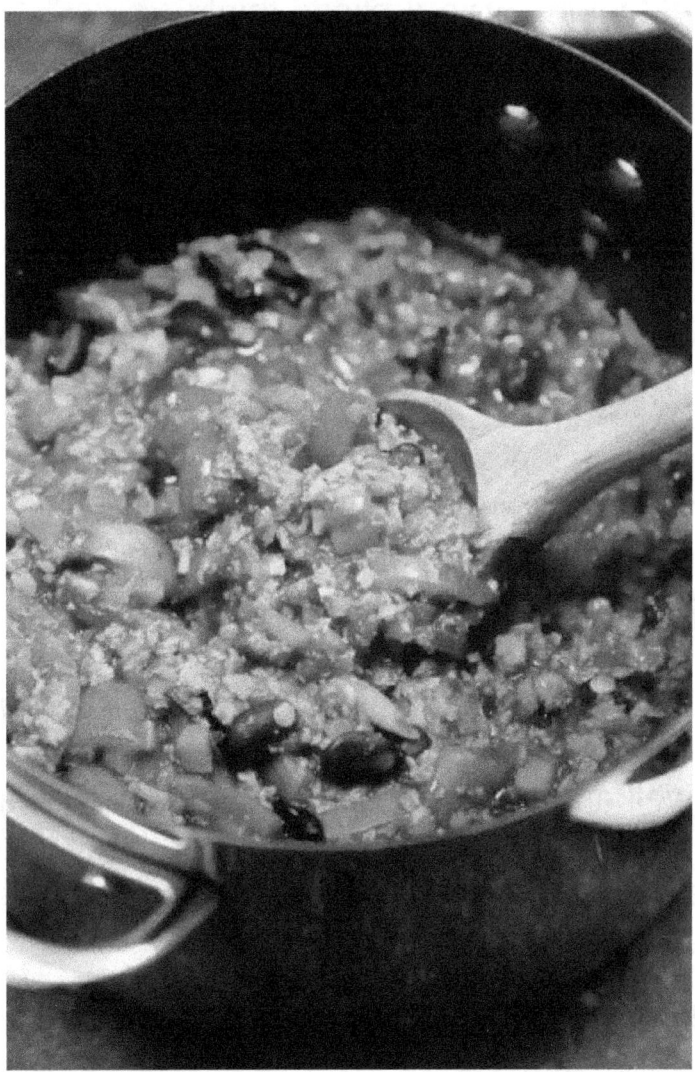

Preparation Time: 10 Minutes
Cooking Time: 30 Minutes
Skill: Beginner
Serving Size: 6

INGREDIENTS:

- 1 tsp. Cumin, ground
- 3 Garlic cloves, minced
- 1 tsp. Chili Powder
- 2 tbsp. Olive Oil
- 2 Carrots, medium & finely chopped

- 2 Celery Stalks, finely chopped
- ½ cup Vegetable Stock
- 1 Red Onion, large & sliced thinly
- Salt & Pepper, as needed
- 14 oz. Soy Mince, frozen
- 2 Red Peppers, finely chopped
- 14 oz. Red Kidney Beans, washed & drained
- 3 ½ oz. Split Red Lentils
- 1 ¾ lb. Chopped Tomatoes

COOKING INSTRUCTIONS:

- To make this highly satiating meal, you need to first heat a large saucepan over a medium heat.
- Spoon in the oil and once the oil becomes hot, stir in the peppers, garlic, carrots, celery, and tomatoes.
- Sauté for 2 to 3 minutes or until the veggies are soft.
- Next, spoon in the cumin, pepper, chili powder, and salt to the pan.
- Mix well and then add kidney beans, vegetable stock, chopped tomatoes, soy mince, and lentil to the mixture.
- Give a gentle stir and allow it to simmer for 20 to 25 minutes.
- Serve it hot.

Tip: For more flavor, you can try adding miso paste.

NUTRITIONAL INFORMATION PER SERVING:

- Calories: 340 Kcal
- Protein: 25g
- Carbohydrates: 42g
- Fat: 2g

VEGAN TOFU SPINACH LASAGNE

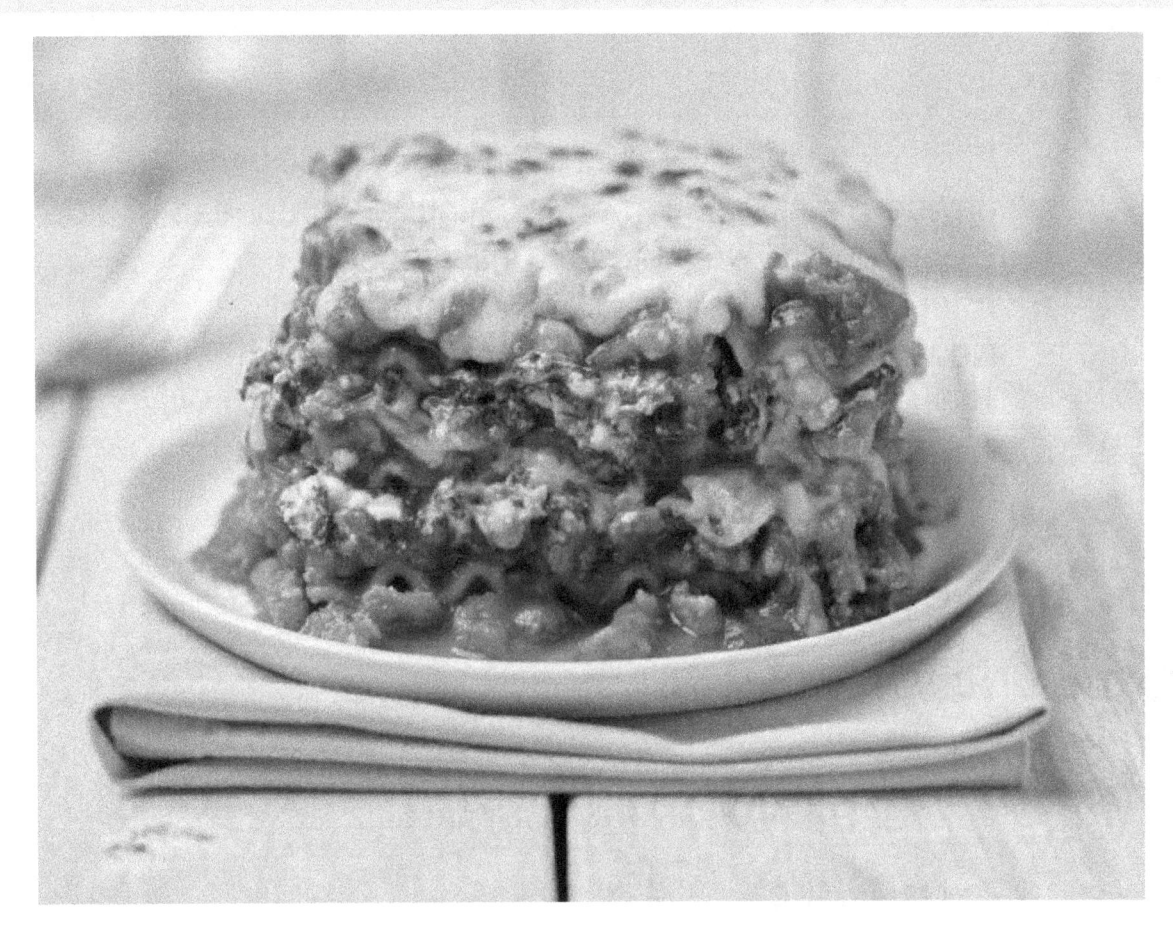

Preparation Time: 10 Minutes
Cooking Time: 15 Minutes
Skill: Beginner
Serving Size: 6

INGREDIENTS:

- 10 oz. Lasagne
- 20 oz. Bag of Spinach, thawed
- 14 oz. Tofu, firm
- 4 cups Tomato Sauce
- 1 tsp. Salt
- ¼ cup Soy Milk
- ½ tsp. Garlic Powder
- 2 tbsp. Lime Juice

- 10 oz. Lasagne Noodles
- 3 tbsp. Basil, fresh & chopped

COOKING INSTRUCTIONS:

- First, place the tofu along with the soy milk, salt, garlic powder, basil, and lemon juice into a high-speed blender.
- Blend for 1 to 2 minutes or until smooth.
- After that, stir in the spinach and mash well.
- Now, pour the tomato sauce into the pot.
- Then, layer 1/3 of the lasagne noodles, the spinach mixture, and 1/3 of the tofu on top of it.
- Repeat the layers.
- Next, cook for 6 to 8 hours in the slow cooker.
- Serve it hot.

Tip: If desired, you can add basil leaves to it.

NUTRITIONAL INFORMATION PER SERVING:

- Calories: 284Kcal
- Protein: 20.1 g
- Carbohydrates: 42g
- Fat: 5.9g

SESAME TOFU WITH SOBA NOODLES

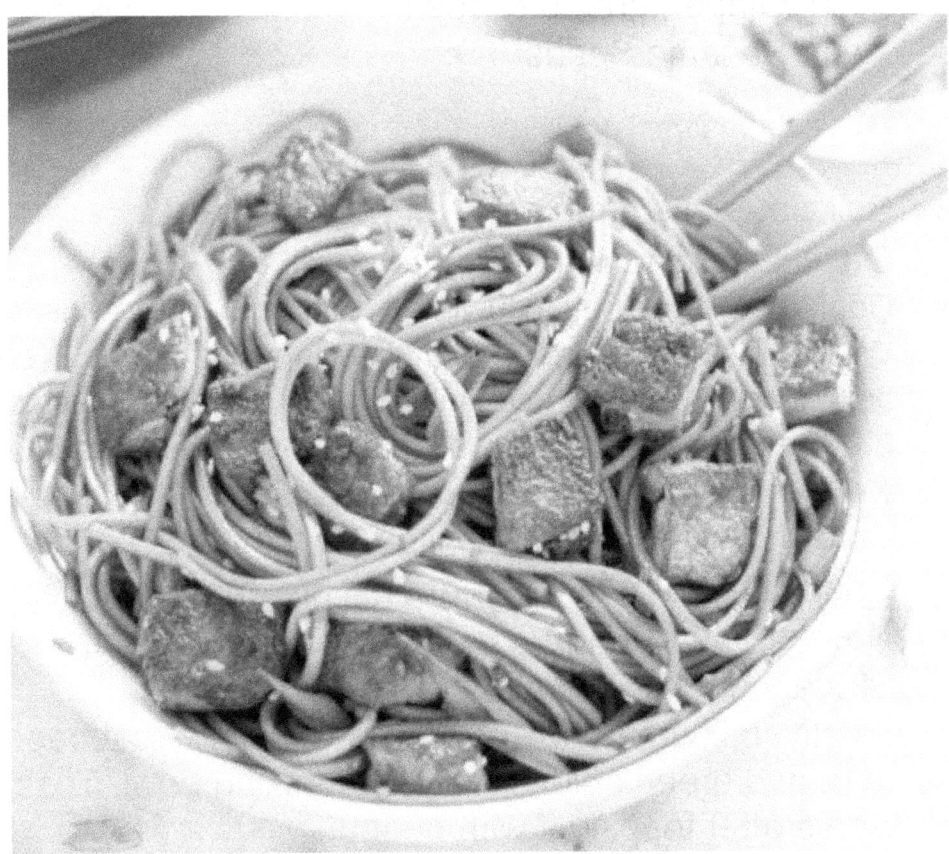

Preparation Time: 10 Minutes
Cooking Time: 15 Minutes
Skill: Beginner
Serving Size: 4

INGREDIENTS:

- 2 cups Cabbage, shredded
- 1 lb. Soba
- 14 oz. Tofu, firm & cubed
- 2 Green Onions, thinly sliced
- 2 tbsp. Soy Sauce
- ¼ cup Rice Vinegar
- 1 Garlic clove, crushed
- 1 tbsp. Sesame Oil
- 2 Green Onions, thinly sliced
- 2 tsp. Brown Sugar

- Peanuts, crushed, for garnishing
- 1 tsp. Vegetable Oil
- 1 tsp. Ginger, grated & fresh
- 1 tsp. Sesame Seeds

COOKING INSTRUCTIONS:

- Boil water in a large pot over medium heat.
- Once it starts boiling, add the noodles.
- Cook the noodles by following the manufacturer's instructions.
- Wash the noodles under cold water and then drain. Keep it
- aside. After that, mix rice vinegar, sesame seeds, soy sauce, brown sugar, and sesame oil in a small bowl until combined
- well. Next, spoon oil in a heated skillet over medium-high heat.
- Once the oil becomes hot, stir in the tofu.
- Cook them for 4 minutes or until browned. Set it aside.
- Now, spoon in ginger, cabbage, and garlic to it,
- Sauté them for 2 minutes or until softened.
- Finally, mix the noodles, rice wine mixture, cabbage, tofu, and green onions in a large mixing bowl. Toss well.
- Serve after topping it with peanuts.

Tip: For a spicier kick, you can use sriracha sauce on the noodles.

NUTRITIONAL INFORMATION PER SERVING:

- Calories: 549Kcal
- Protein: 25.8g
- Carbohydrates: 91.7g
- Fat: 12.2g

MEXICAN GREEN LENTIS SOUP

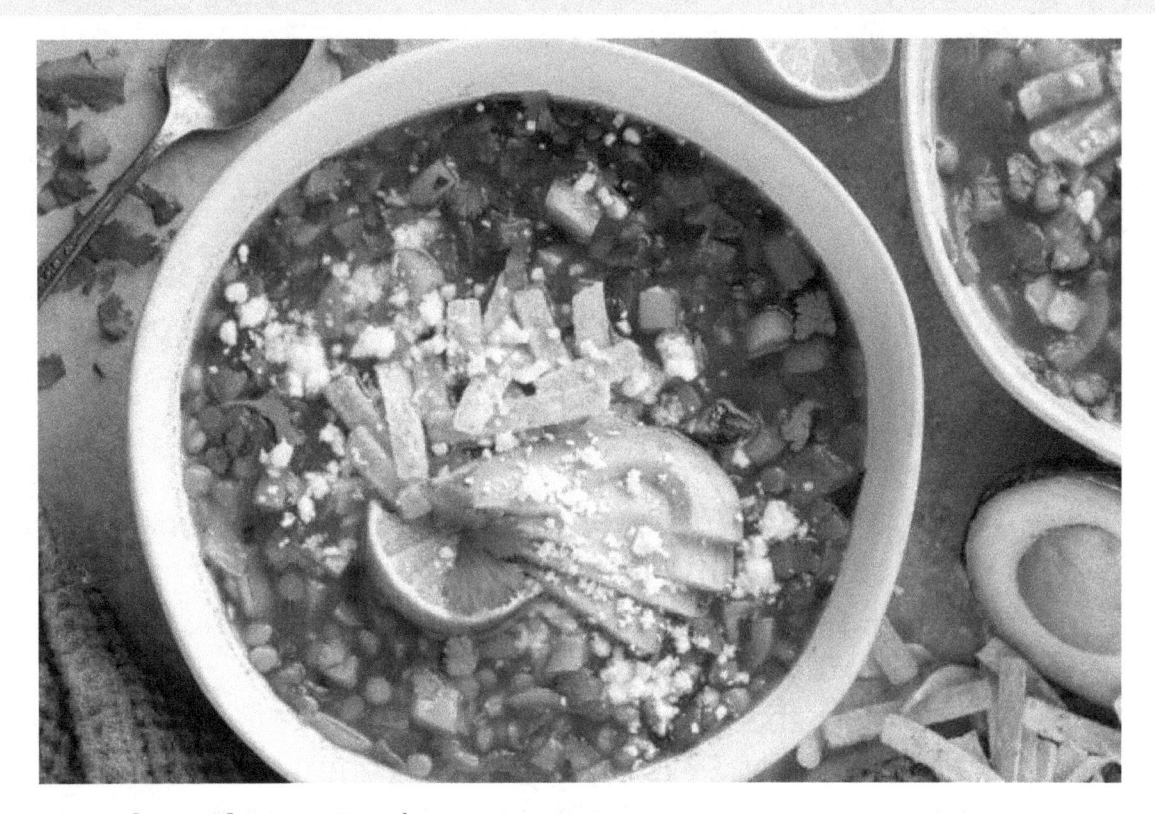

Preparation Time: 10 Minutes
Cooking Time: 45 Minutes
Skill: Beginner
Serving Size: 6

INGREDIENTS:

- 2 cups Green Lentils
- 2 tbsp. Extra Virgin Olive Oil
- 8 oz. can of Diced Tomatoes & Chilies
- 1 Yellow Onion, diced
- ½ tsp. Salt
- 2 Celery Stalks, diced
- 2 Carrots, peeled & diced
- 1 Red Bell Pepper, diced
- 8 cups Vegetable Broth
- 2 cups Diced Tomatoes & Juices
- 3 Garlic cloves, minced

- 1 tsp. Oregano
- 1 tbsp. Cumin
- ¼ tsp. Smoked Paprika
- 1 Avocado, pitted & diced

COOKING INSTRUCTIONS:

- Heat oil in a large-sized pot over a medium heat.
- Once the oil becomes hot, stir in the onion, bell pepper, carrot, and celery into the pot.
- Cook the onion mixture for 5 minutes or until the veggies are soft.
- Then, spoon in garlic, oregano, cumin, and paprika into it and sauté for one minute or until aromatic.
- Next, add the tomatoes, salt, chilies, broth, and lentils to the mixture.
- Now, bring the tomato-chili mixture to a boil and allow it to simmer for 32 to 40 minutes or until the lentils
- become soft. Check the seasoning and add more if
- needed. Serve along with avocado and hot sauce.

Tip: You can avoid onion if you desire.

NUTRITIONAL INFORMATION PER SERVING:

- Calories: 235Kcal
- Protein: 9g
- Carbohydrates: 32g
- Fat: 9g

LEMON FETTUCINE ALFREDO

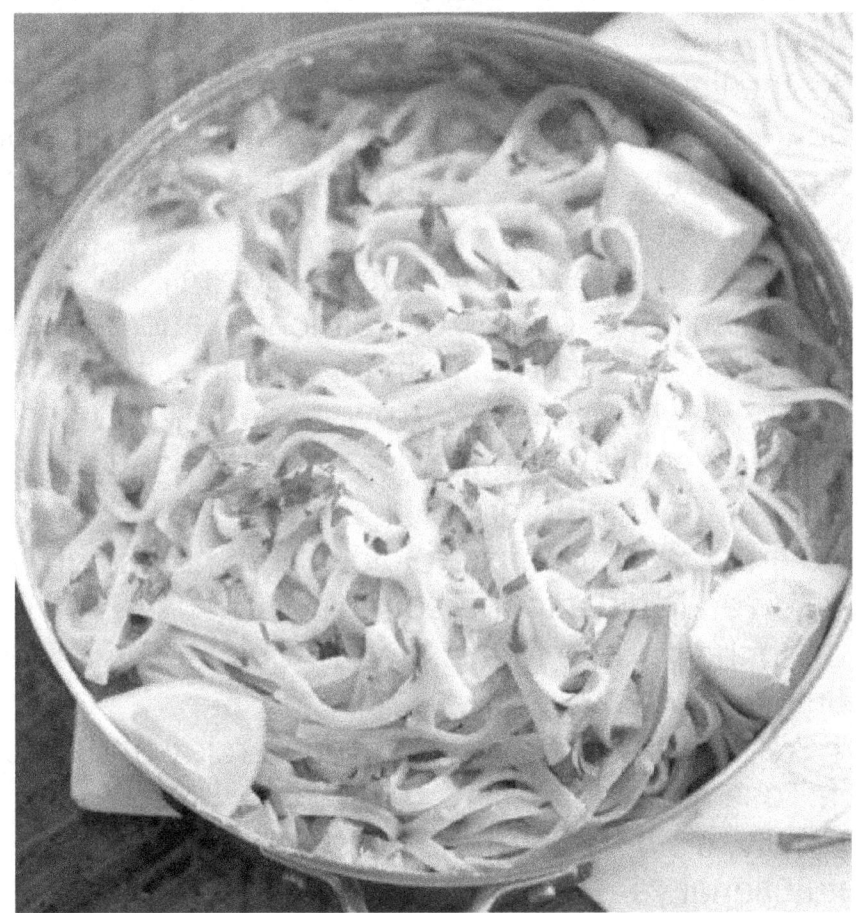

Preparation Time: 10 Minutes
Cooking Time: 35 Minutes
Serving Size: 4

INGREDIENTS:

- ½ cup Parsley leaves, loosely packed &
- chopped 4 oz. Soy Cream Cheese
- 2 tbsp. Extra Virgin Olive Oil
- 2 cups Almond Milk, unsweetened
- 3 Garlic cloves, finely chopped
- 3 tbsp. Nutritional Yeast
- 12 oz. Fettucine, eggless
- Salt & Pepper, as needed
- 3 tbsp. Almonds, blanched & sliced
- 1 tsp. Lemon Zest, finely grated

COOKING INSTRUCTIONS:

- To begin with, heat a large pot over a medium-high heat or until the water is boiling.
- As the liquid starts to boil, stir in the fettuccine and cook al dente by following the instructions given on the packet.
- Drain the cooked pasta and reserve one cup of the cooking liquid.
- Next, stir in the nutritional yeast, soy milk, pepper, soy cream cheese, lemon zest, almonds, and salt into a high-
- speed blender. Blend them for a minute or two or until
- you get a smooth paste. Now, spoon oil into a large
- skillet. When it becomes hot, stir in the garlic.
- Sauté for a minute or until it sizzles.
- Pour the soy milk mixture along with half a cup of the reserved liquid into the pot.
- Bring the mixture to a simmer. Cook for 8 minutes or until thickened.
- Take the pot from the heat. Add parsley and fettuccine to it. Toss well.
- Finally, divide among the balls and top it with the nutritional yeast.

Tip: Instead of soy milk, you can also use almond milk.

NUTRITIONAL INFORMATION PER SERVING:

- Calories: 520Kcal
- Protein: 22g
- Carbohydrates: 74g
- Fat: 15g

QUINOA BOWLS WITH SPIRALIZED ZUCCHINI

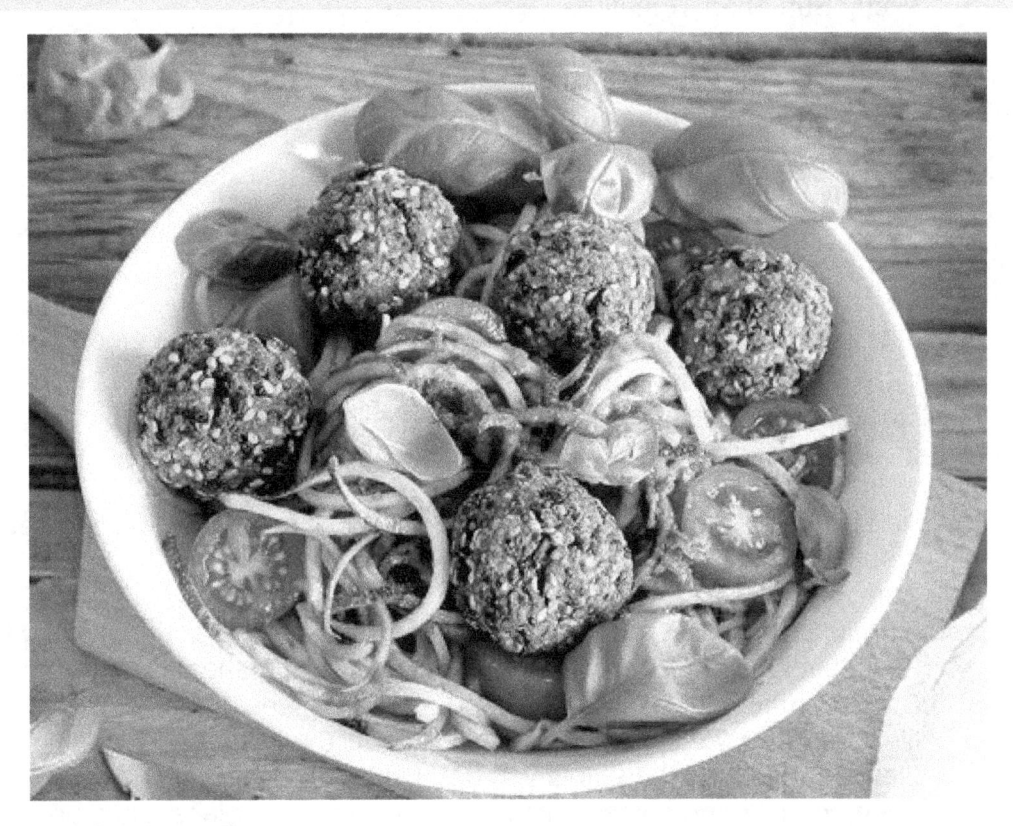

Preparation Time: 10 Minutes
Cooking Time: 45 Minutes
Skill: Beginner
Serving Size: 6

INGREDIENTS:

- 4 Zucchini

For the balls:

- ½ cup Quinoa
- 1 ½ tbsp. Herbs, fresh
- 2 tbsp. Tomato Paste
- 14 oz. can of Black Beans
- ½ tbsp. Sriracha
- 1 tsp. Garlic Powder
- ¼ cup Sesame Seeds
- 2 tbsp. Nutritional Yeast
- ¼ cup Oat Flour

For the sun-dried tomato sauce:

- 1 tbsp. Apple Cider Vinegar
- ½ cup Cherry Tomatoes, halved
- ½ cup Sun-dried Tomatoes
- 1 tsp. Oregano
- 1 Garlic clove
- 2 tbsp. Pine Nuts, toasted
- A handful of Basil, fresh
- 2 tbsp. Nutritional Yeast

COOKING INSTRUCTIONS:

- First, place quinoa and a cup of water in a deep saucepan over a medium heat.
- Cook the grains for 13 to 15 minutes.
- Once cooked, drain away the water and allow the rice to cool.
- In the meantime, put the black beans into a large mixing bowl and mash with a potato masher.
- Add the cooked quinoa, tomato paste, oat flour, sriracha, sesame seeds, tomato paste, and seasoning.
- Combine the mixture until you get a smooth dough.
- Now, use two tablespoon-sized scoops of the mixture and make into balls.
- Place the balls on a parchment paper-lined baking sheet.
- Bake them at 400° F or 200 °C for 38 to 40 minutes or until crispy.
- Next, to make the sun-dried sauce, place all the ingredients in a high-speed blender and blend them until you get a smooth paste.
- Then, to make the pasta, spiralize the zucchini and place it in a bowl.
- Finally, add the tomato sauce and the balls to the pasta and toss well.
- Garnish it with basil and serve.

Tip: If desired, you can add basil leaves to it.

NUTRITIONAL INFORMATION PER SERVING:

- Calories: 235Kcal
- Protein: 9g
- Carbohydrates: 32g
- Fat: 9g

SWEET & SOUR TEMPEH

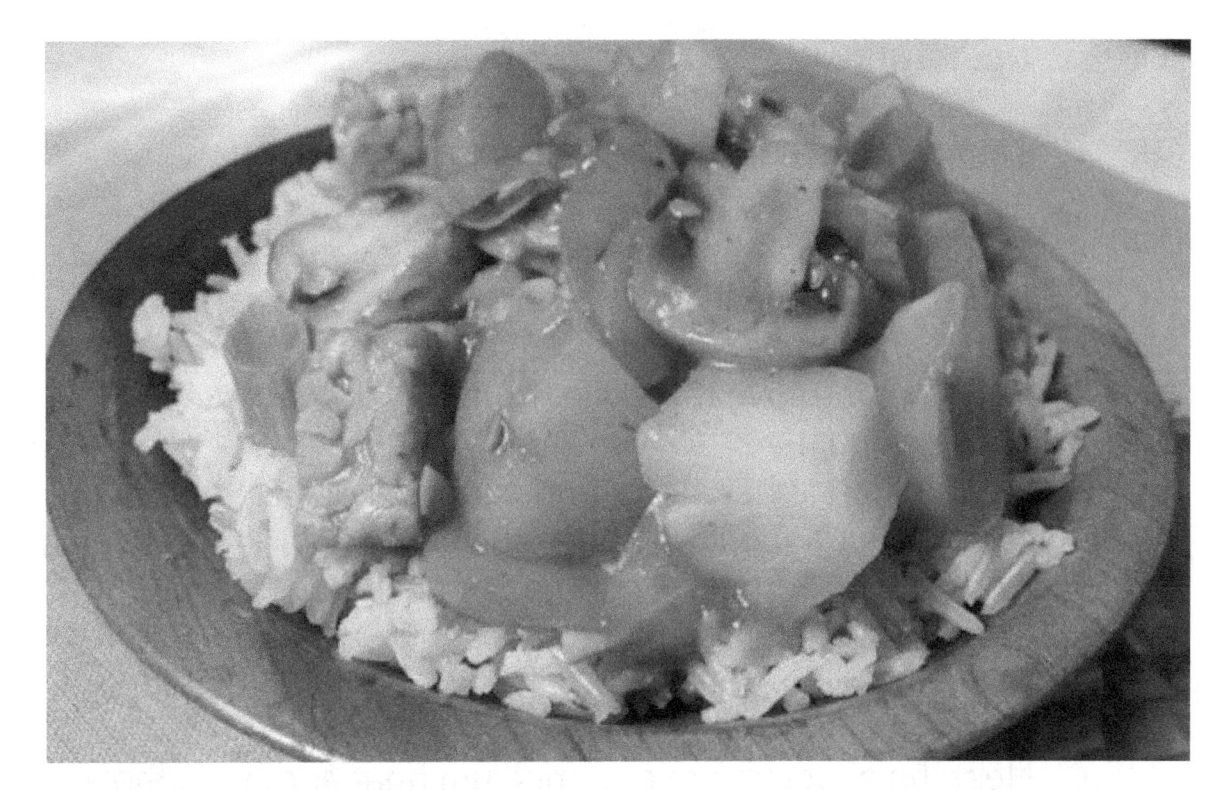

Preparation Time: 10 Minutes
Cooking Time: 30 Minutes
Skill: Beginner
Serving Size: 3

INGREDIENTS:

- 1o oz. Tempeh
- 2 tbsp. Olive Oil
- 2 tbsp. Soy Sauce
- ¾ cup Vegetable Broth

For the sauce:

- 1 tbsp. Cornstarch
- 15 oz. Pineapple Chunks
- 1 Yellow Onion, chopped
- 1 cup mushrooms, diced
- ¼ cup Vinegar
- 2 tbsp. Brown Sugar
- 1 Red Bell Pepper, chopped

COOKING INSTRUCTIONS:

- To make this delightful fare, heat a large skillet over a medium-high heat.
- Next, place the tempeh along with the vegetable broth and soy sauce in it.
- Braise the tempeh for about 8 to 10 minutes or until soft.
- After that, remove the skillet from the heat and keep the braising liquid.
- Now, take another skillet and spoon olive oil into it.
- Heat it over a medium heat and stir in the braised tempeh.
- Cook the mixture for 3 minutes or until browned.
- In the meantime, to make the sauce combine the reserved pineapple juice, vinegar, cornstarch and brown sugar in a saucepan.
- Heat the saucepan over a medium heat and bring the mixture to a simmer while stirring it continuously.
- Then, add the onion, mushrooms, and pepper to it and continue stirring until the mixture thickens.
- Finally, lower the heat and stir in the braised tempeh and pineapple chunks and simmer for
- another 5 minutes. Serve it hot.

Tip: Pair it with couscous or another whole grain.

NUTRITIONAL INFORMATION PER SERVING:

- Calories: 309Kcal
- Protein: 10 g
- Carbohydrates: 41g
- Fat: 13g

DESSERTS FOR A GOOD MOOD

VANILLA CHIA QUINOA PUDDING

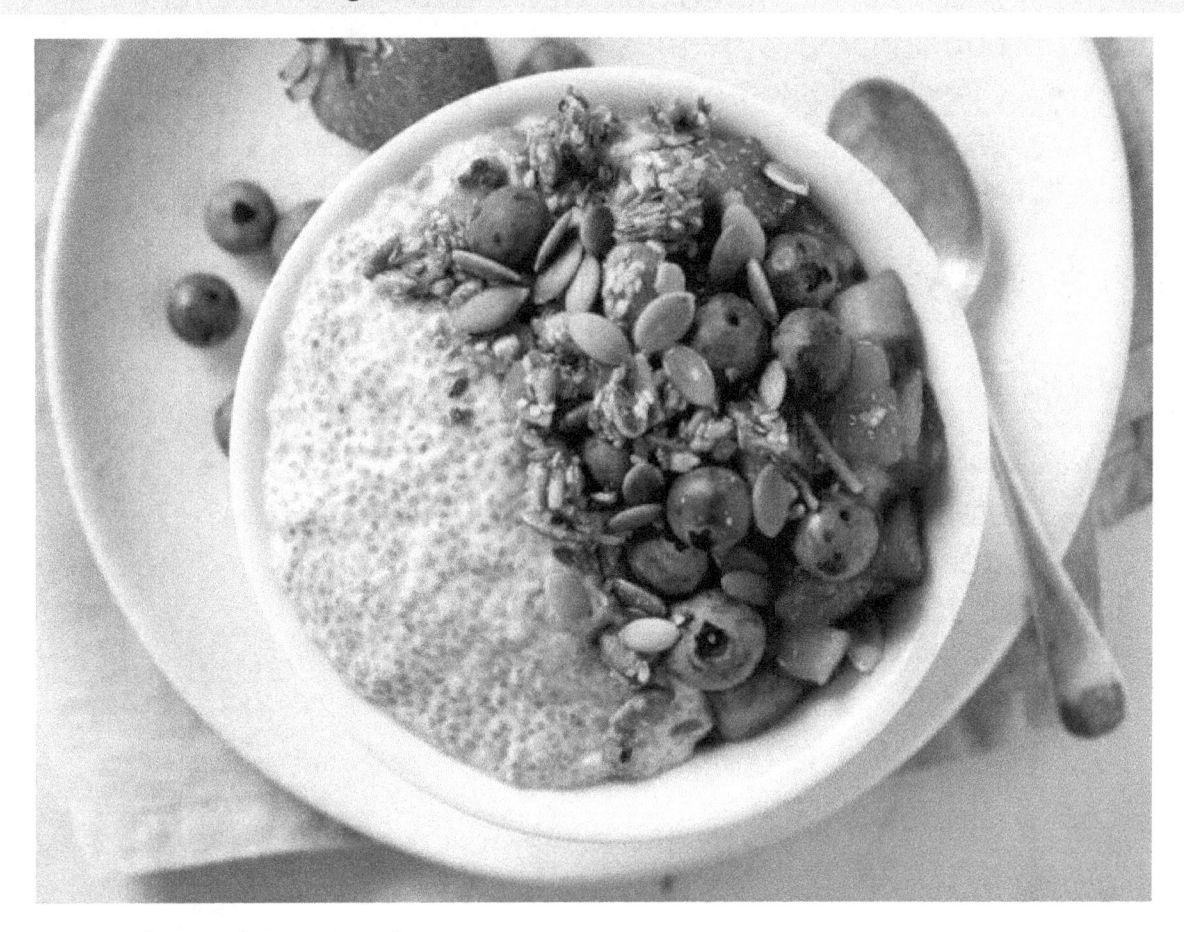

Preparation Time: 5 Minutes
Cooking Time: 10 Minutes
Skill: Beginner
Serving Size: 1

INGREDIENTS:

- 2 tbsp. Chia Seeds
- ¾ cup Cashew Milk
- ¼ tsp. Vanilla
- ¼ cup Quinoa, cooked
- Dash of Cinnamon
- 2 tbsp. Hemp Seeds

- 2 tbsp. Maple Syrup

COOKING INSTRUCTION:

- Place all the ingredients needed to make the breakfast pudding in a large mason jar and combine well.
- Close the lid. Keep the jar in the refrigerator for at least 2 hours or until set.
- Serve and enjoy.

Tip: If desired, you can top it with toppings like berries or seeds, etc.

NUTRITIONAL INFORMATION PER SERVING:

- Calories: 258 Kcal
- Protein: 16g
- Carbohydrates: 13g
- Fat: 13g

CHOCOLATE CHIA PUDDING

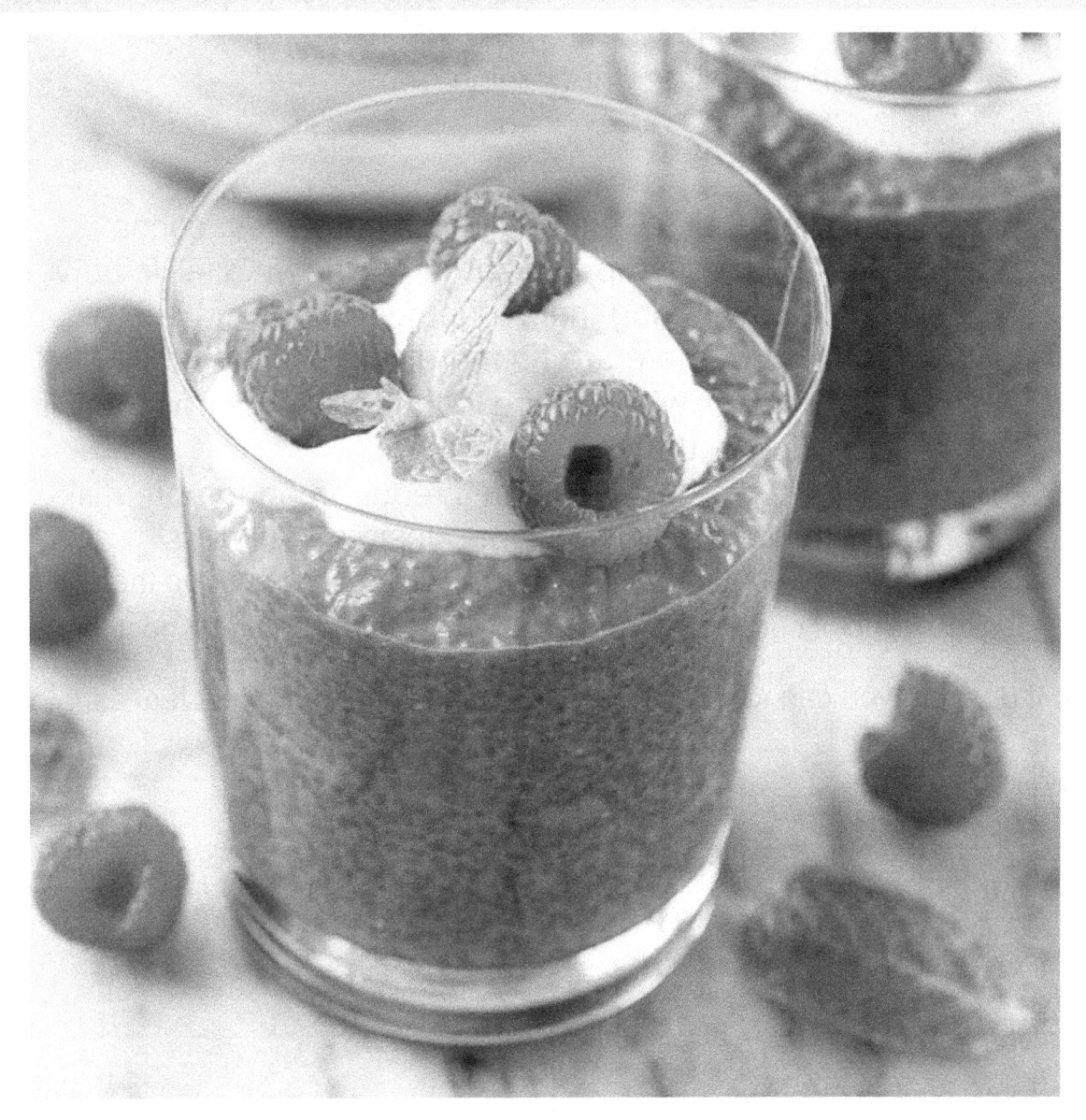

Preparation Time: 15 Minutes
Cooking Time: 2 to 6 hours in the refrigerator
Skill: Beginner
Serving Size: 2

INGREDIENTS:

- ¼ cup Chia seeds
- 1 tbsp. Cocoa powder

- 1 tbsp. Pure Maple syrup
- 1½ cup unsweetened Almond Milk or as required to dilute
- 2 tbsp. Carob powder
- Shaved chocolate, for garnish

COOKING INSTRUCTIONS:

- To start with, place almond milk, chia seeds, cocoa powder, maple syrup and carob powder in a large bowl. Then, start whisking them together and continue the whisking until there are no more clumps in the mixture.
- Place the bowl with mixture in the refrigerator and chill it for 2 hours or for overnight.
- After that, stir them well and if required pour more milk to the mixture to achieve your desired thickness.
- Serve the pudding in individual serving bowls and top them with a dollop of coconut cream. Garnish it with the shaved chocolate.

Tip: If desired, you can top it with toppings like berries and mint leaves, etc.

NUTRITIONAL INFORMATION PER SERVING:

- Calories: 258 Kcal
- Proteins: 16g
- Carbohydrates: 13g
- Fat: 13g

BANANA PEANUT BUTTER OATMEAL

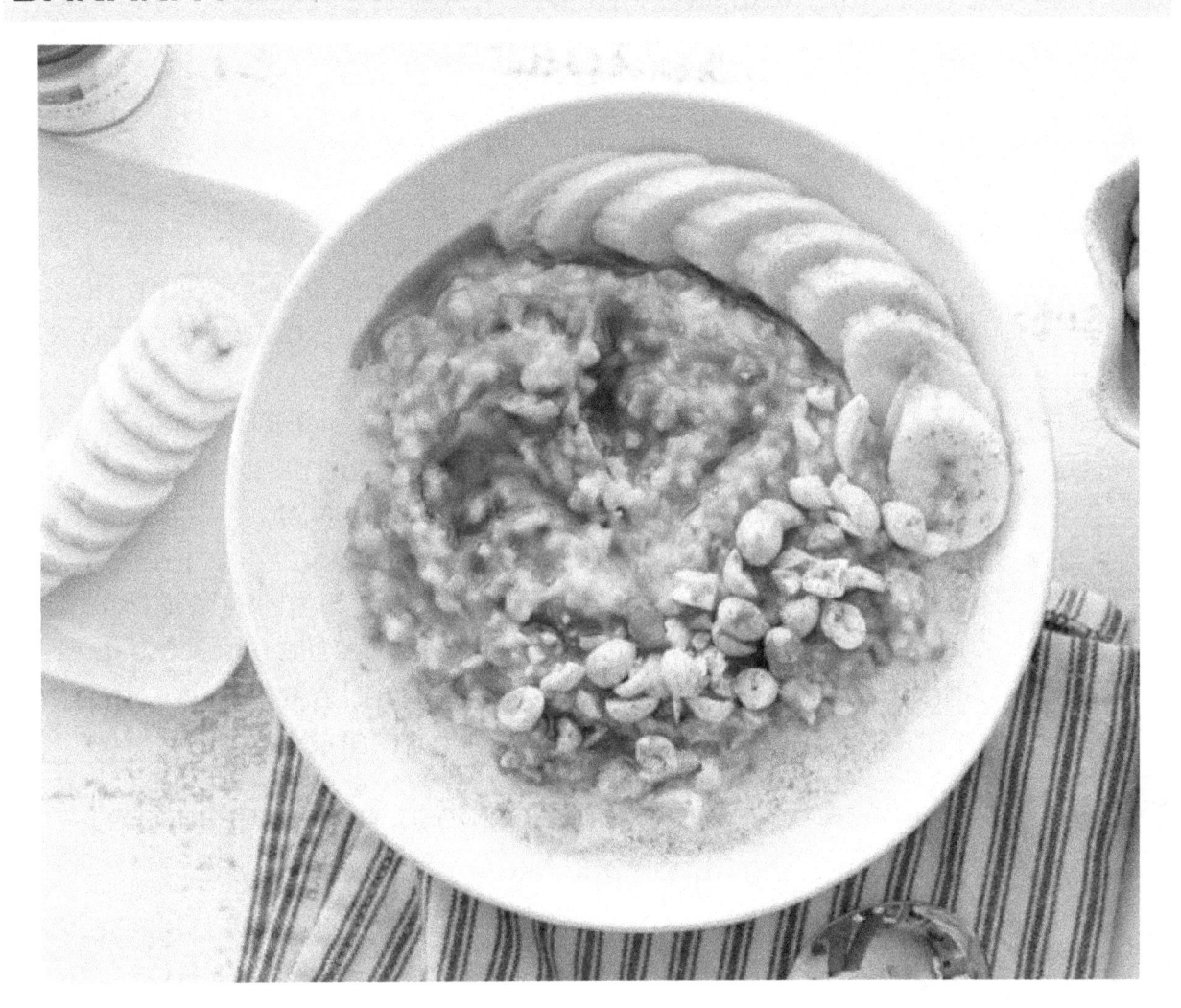

Preparation Time: 5 Minutes
Cooking Time: 35 Minutes
Skill: Beginner
Serving Size: 2

INGREDIENTS:

- ½ cup rolled Oats
- ½ tbsp. Natural Peanut Butter
- 1 large very ripe Banana
- ½ to 1 tsp. Chia seed or flax seeds
- 1 cup Almond Milk
- 1 tsp. Non-dairy Butter (or Coconut Oil)

- ¼ tsp. Ground Nutmeg
- 1 tsp. Pure Vanilla Extract
- 1 tsp. Ground Cinnamon
- Pinch of salt

COOKING INSTRUCTIONS:

- First, you need to peel and chop the banana in large
- pieces. Now, heat a medium-sized pot over medium heat and then cook the banana and non-dairy butter for about 5 minutes while stirring frequently.
- Add ½ tbsp. of peanut butter and after that, stir in the oats, chia seeds, milk, spices, and a pinch of salt to the banana mixture. Beat them together until you get a homogeneous mass.
- Bring the banana mixture to a low boil and then lower the heat. Simmer it for 8 to 10 min while stirring often. Remove the pot from the heat and finally add the vanilla extract to it.
- Add spoon the oatmeal into a bowl and garnish it with peanut butter, nuts, cinnamon, and maple syrup.

Tip: If desired, you can use for toppings 1/2 tbsp. of peanut butter, pure maple syrup, nuts, cinnamon and like banana slices, etc.

NUTRITIONAL INFORMATION PER SERVING:

- Calories: 364 Kcal
- Proteins: 19.1g
- Carbohydrates: 32.6g
- Fat: 19g

PUMPKIN PIE PUDDING

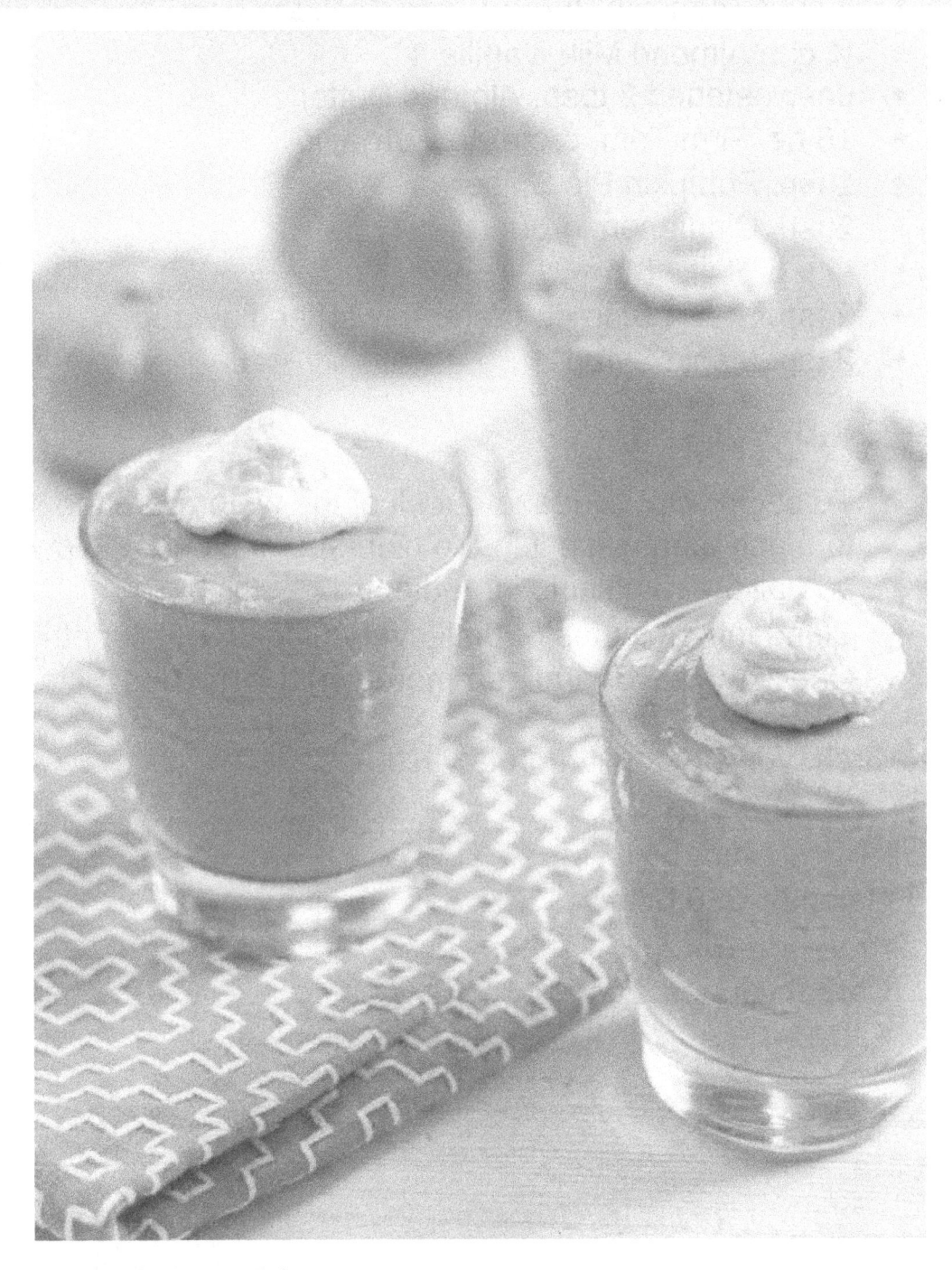

Preparation Time: 10 Minutes
Cooking Time: 20 Minutes
Skill: Beginner
Serving Size: 4

INGREDIENTS:

- 2 cups Pumpkin Puree
- ¼ cup Almond Milk, vanilla &
- unsweetened 2 tbsp. Almond Butter
- 16 oz. Firm Tofu, preferably organic
- 1 tsp. Pumpkin Pie Spice
- 2 tsp. Cinnamon, ground
- ¼ tsp. Salt
- 2 tsp. Stevia Extract, preferably toffee flavored
- 2 tsp. Maple Syrup

COOKING INSTRUCTION:

- To begin with, squeeze out all of the water from the tofu and then place it in the high-speed blender. Now,
- add all the remaining ingredients.
- Blend for 2 minutes or until everything comes together.
- Check the flavor and add more sugar if needed.

Tip: If desired, you can top it more sweetness.

NUTRITIONAL INFORMATION PER SERVING:

- Calories: 250 Kcal
- Protein: 17g
- Carbohydrates: 20g
- Fat: 11g

BANANA CACAO ICE CREAM

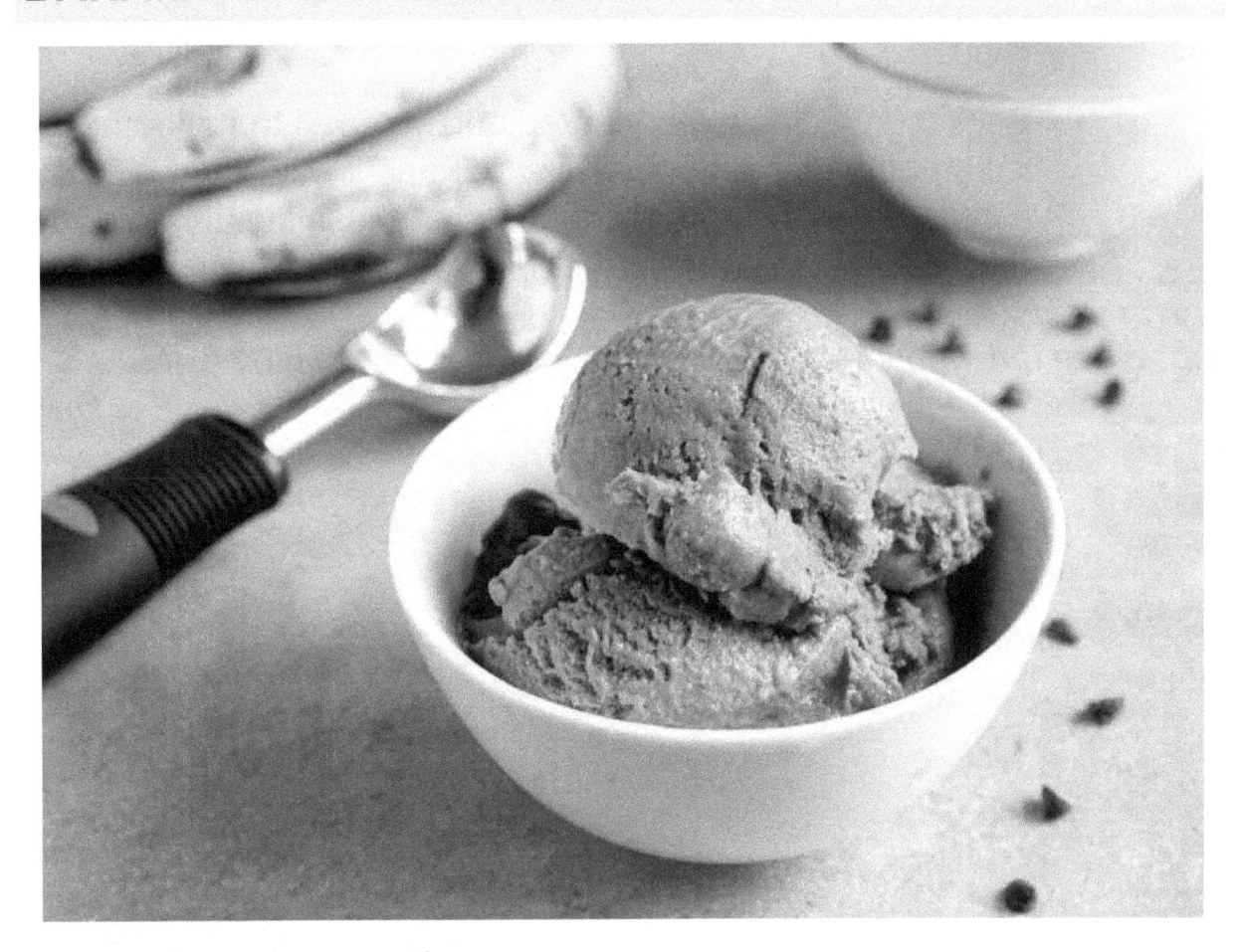

Preparation Time: 5 Minutes
Cooking Time: 10 Minutes
Skill: Beginner
Serving Size: 4

INGREDIENTS:

- 2 Banana, frozen
- 2 tsp. Peanut Butter, natural
- 1 tsp. Maple Syrup
- 1 tbsp. Cacao Powder, raw
- 2 tbsp. Almond Milk
- Dash of Cinnamon
- 1 tsp. Maca Powder
- Chia Seeds, as needed, for garnish

- Flax Seeds, as needed, for garnish

COOKING INSTRUCTION:

- Begin by placing all the ingredients needed to make the ice cream in a high-speed blender and blend them for 2 minutes or until you get a smooth and luscious mixture. After that, transfer to a bowl and top it with chia and flax seeds.

Tip: If desired, you can top it with toppings like cacao nibs also.

NUTRITIONAL INFORMATION PER SERVING:

- Calories: 475 Kcal
- Protein: 33g
- Carbohydrates: 72g
- Fat: 10g

HIGH-PROTEIN SMOOTHIE

BERRY RECOVERY PROTEIN SMOOTHIE

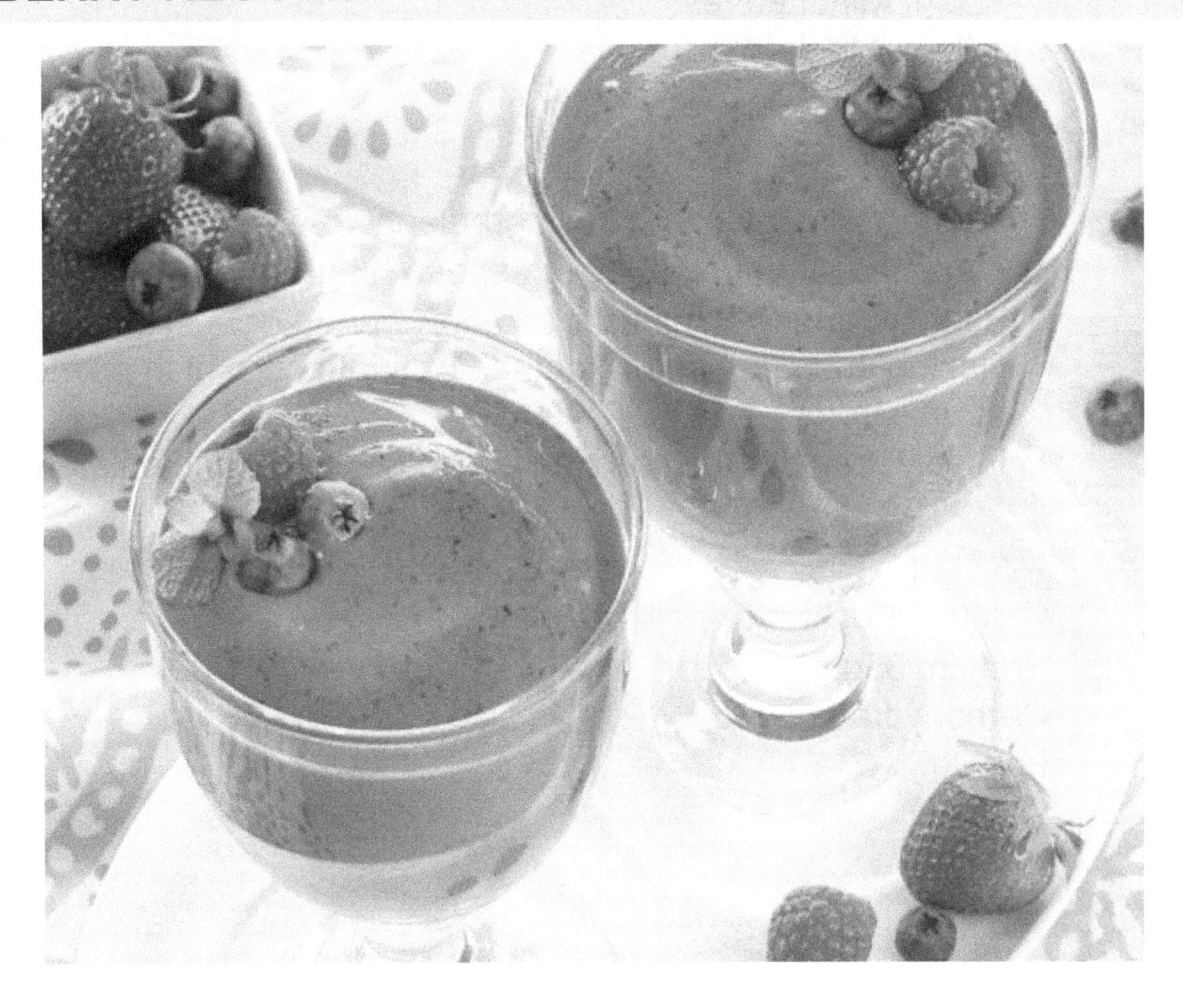

Preparation Time: 5 Minutes
Cooking Time: 5 Minutes
Skill: Beginner
Serving Size: 2

INGREDIENTS:

- 1/2 cup Frozen Mixed Berries (blueberries, raspberries, strawberries, blueberries, etc.)
- 1 cup Vanilla Soy Milk
- 1 Banana, frozen

- 1/2 cup Almond milk
- 2 tbsp. of Protein Powder
- 1tbsp. Flaxseed
- ½ tsp. Mint Leaves
- 1 tbsp. Maple Syrup

COOKING INSTRUCTION:

- To start with, place all the ingredients needed to make the smoothie in a high-speed blender.
- Blend it for 2 to 3 minutes on a low speed or until smooth.
- Next, blend it again for another 1 minute on a high speed or until frothy.
- Finally, transfer to a serving glass and serve immediately.

NUTRITIONAL INFORMATION PER SERVING:

- Calories: 313 Kcal
- Protein: 35g
- Carbohydrates: 30g
- Fat: 9g

GREEN HIGH PROTEIN SMOOTHIE

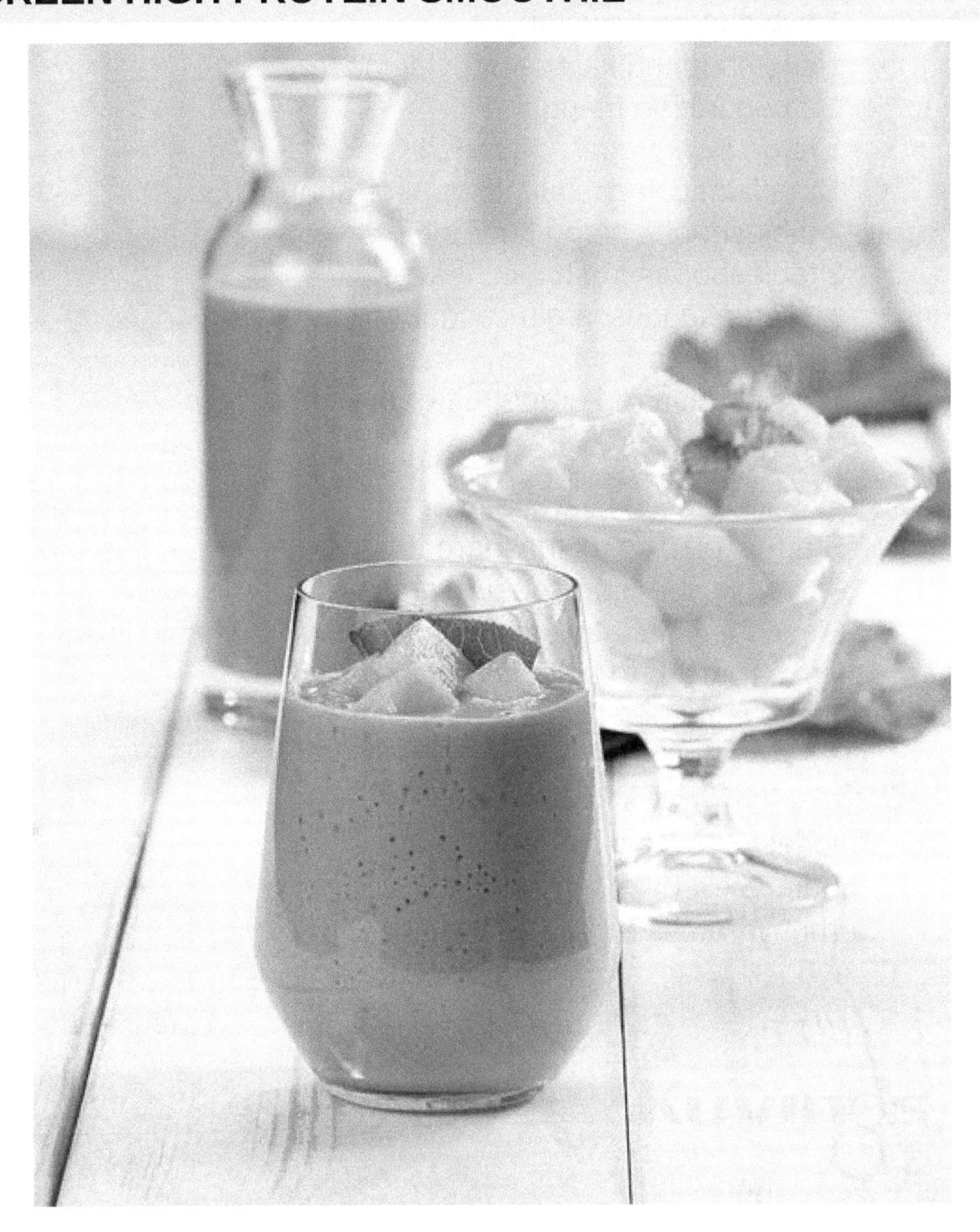

Preparation Time: 5 Minutes
Cooking Time: 5 Minutes
Skill: Beginner
Serving Size: 2

INGREDIENTS:

- 1 cup chopped cucumber
- 1 cup chopped kale or baby spinach
- 1/3 cup frozen mango
- 1 large sweet apple chopped
- 1 medium celery stalk, chopped (about 1/2 cup)
- 2 tablespoons hemp hearts
- 2 tablespoons fresh mint leaves
- 1 1/2 teaspoons virgin coconut oil (optional)
- 4-5 ice cubes
- 1/2 cup fresh red grapefruit or orange juice

COOKING INSTRUCTION:

- Start by placing all the ingredients needed to make the smoothie in a high-speed blender.
- Blend them for 1 to 2 minutes or until smooth and luxurious.
- Next, transfer to a serving glass
- Serve immediately and enjoy.

NUTRITIONAL INFORMATION PER SERVING:

- Calories: 345 Kcal
- Protein: 55g
- Carbohydrates: 20g
- Fat: 8g

BANANA MANGO SMOOTHIE

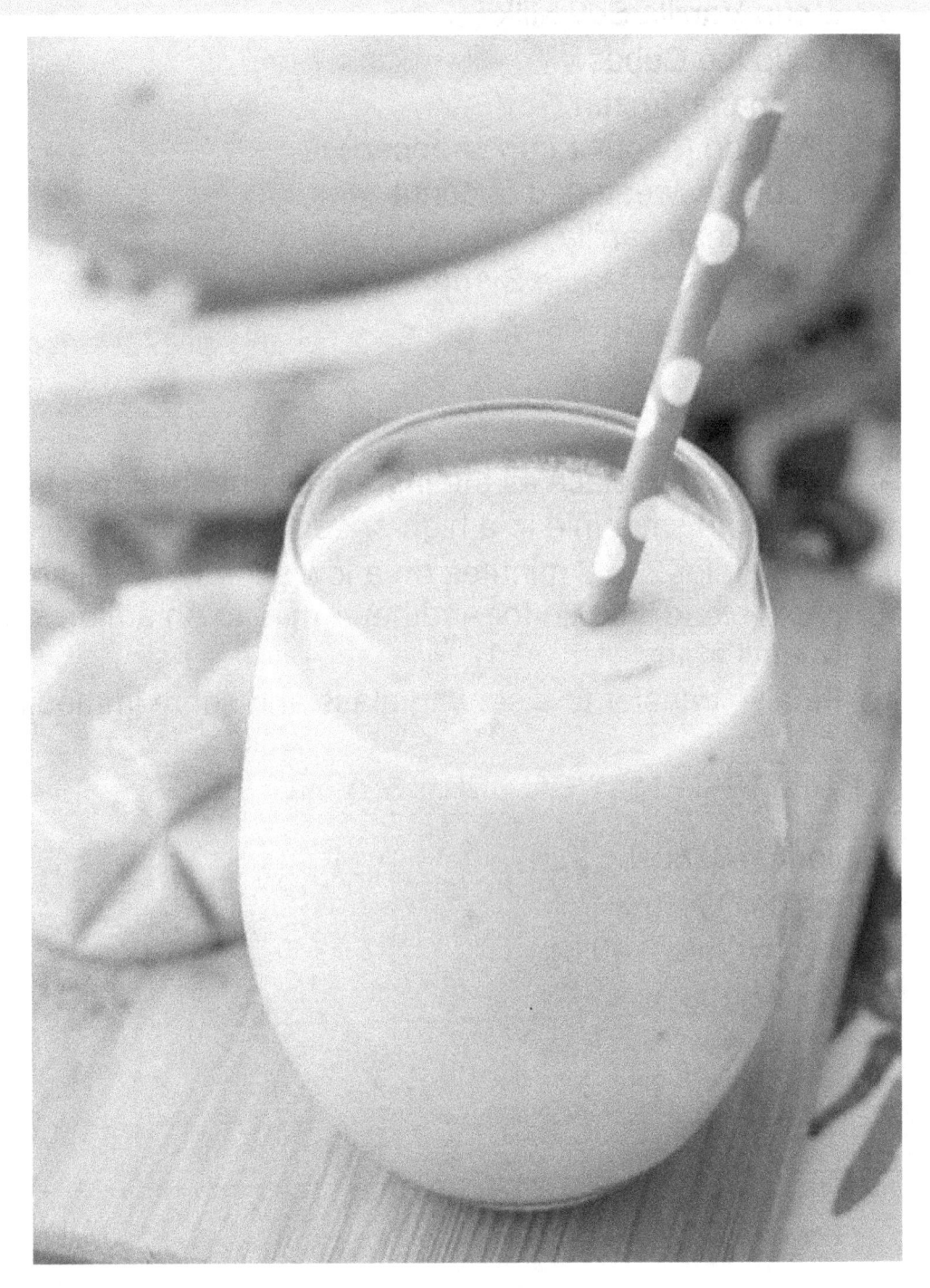

Preparation Time: 5 Minutes
Cooking Time: 5 Minutes
Skill: Beginner
Serving Size: 2

INGREDIENTS:

- 1 cup Vanilla Soy Milk
- 1 cup Ice Cubes
- 1 Banana, frozen
- 1 Mango (about 1 cup chopped)
- ⅛ cup unsweetened coconut
- 1 teaspoon vanilla
- 1 tablespoon Maple Syrup
- 1 tbsp. Chia Seeds

COOKING INSTRUCTION:

- To start with, place all the ingredients needed to make the smoothie in a high-speed blender.
- Blend it for 2 to 3 minutes on a low speed or until smooth.
- Next, blend it again for another 1 minute on a high speed or until frothy.
- Finally, transfer to a serving glass and serve immediately.

NUTRITIONAL INFORMATION PER SERVING:

- Calories: 328cal
- Proteins: 17.4g
- Carbohydrates: 40.8g
- Fat: 12.5g

BANANA AVOCADO AND HEMPSEED SMOOTHIE

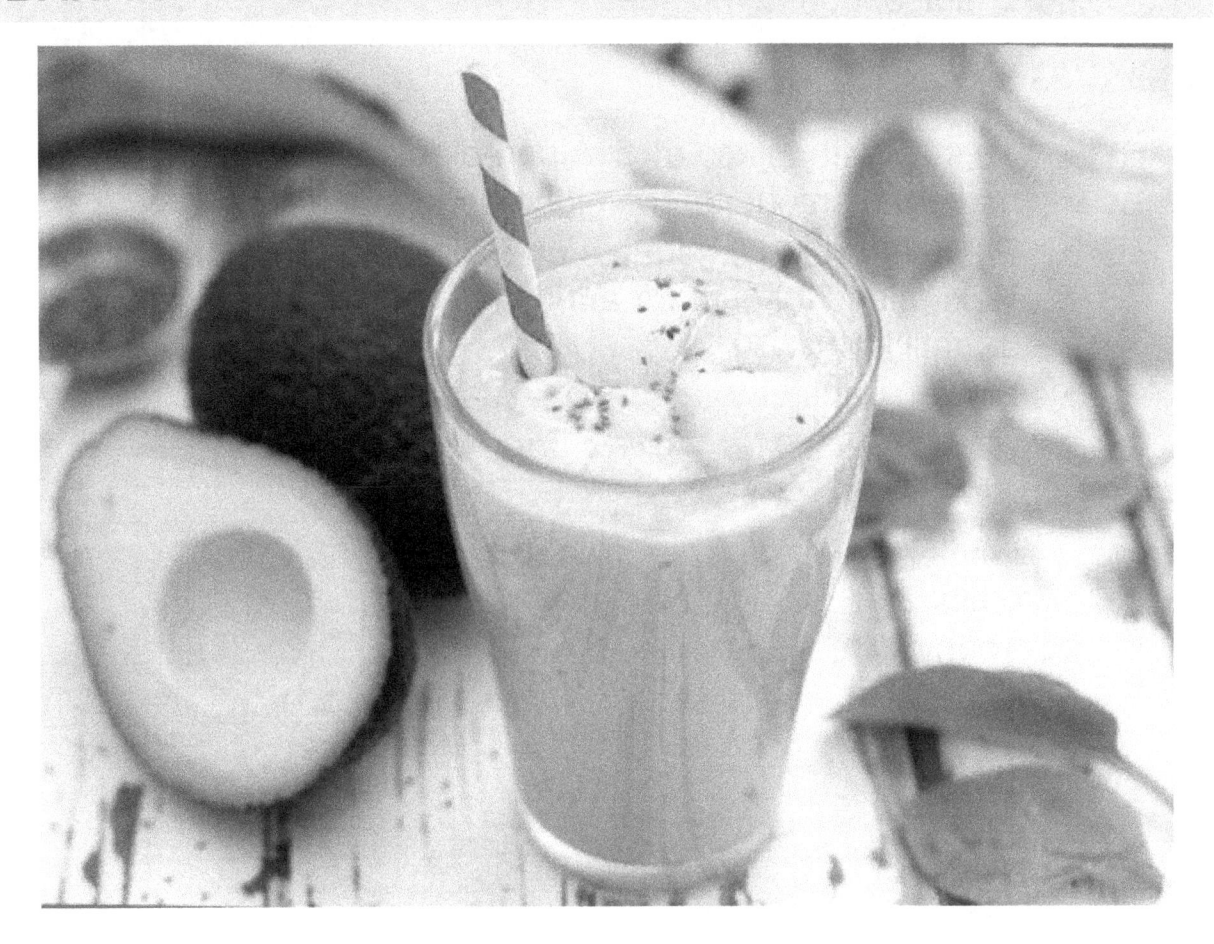

Preparation Time: 5 Minutes
Cooking Time: 5 Minutes
Skill: Beginner
Serving Size: 2

INGREDIENTS:

- 1/2 large avocado
- 1 ripe banana, frozen
- 1 ripe pear, peeled
- 1 sweet apple, chopped
- 1/4 cup parsley
- 1 cup Kale or greens of choice (spinach, collards, and chard)
- 1 1/4 cups almond milk

- 1 teaspoon lemon juice
- 1 tablespoon hemp seeds

COOKING INSTRUCTION:

- To start with, place all the ingredients needed to make the smoothie in a high-speed blender.
- Blend it for 2 to 3 minutes on a low speed or until smooth.
- Next, blend it again for another 1 minute on a high speed or until frothy.
- Finally, transfer to a serving glass and serve immediately.

NUTRITIONAL INFORMATION PER SERVING:

- Calories: 315 Kcal
- Protein: 35g
- Carbohydrates: 25g
- Fat: 10g

BANANA STRAWBERRY CHIA SMOOTHIE

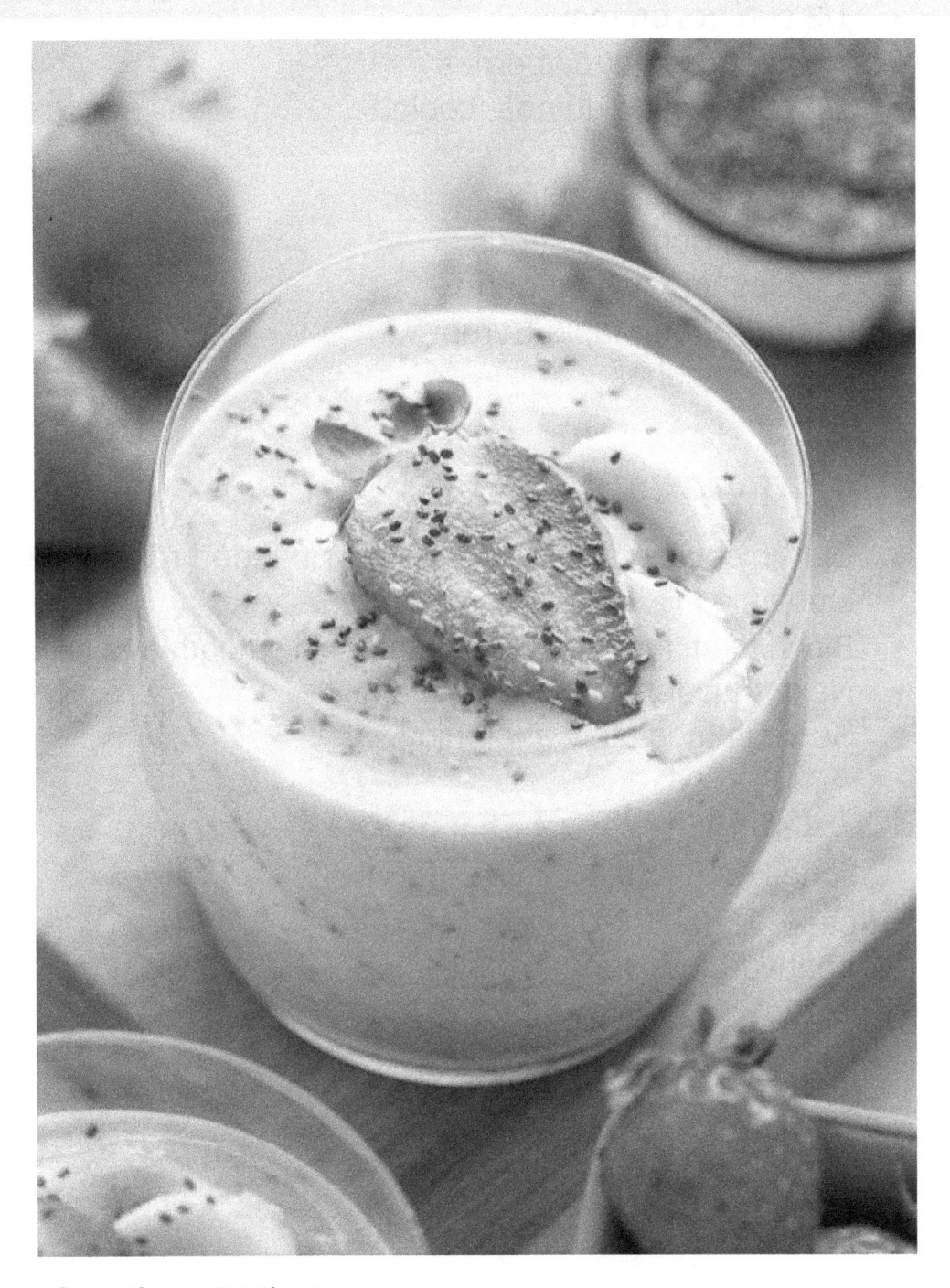

Preparation Time: 5 Minutes
Cooking Time: 5 Minutes
Skill: Beginner
Serving Size: 2

INGREDIENTS:

- 1/3 cup frozen mango
- 1 cups frozen strawberries
- 1/2 cup cooked quinoa, cooled
- 1 large ripe banana
- 2 cup Vanilla Soy Milk
- 1 tablespoon chia seeds
- 1 tablespoon wheat germ
- 2 tablespoon Maple Syrup
- 1 cup ice cubes

COOKING INSTRUCTION:

- Start by placing all the ingredients needed to make the smoothie in a high-speed blender.
- Blend them for 1 to 2 minutes or until smooth and luxurious.
- Next, transfer to a serving glass
- Serve immediately and enjoy.

NUTRITIONAL INFORMATION PER SERVING:

- Calories: 315 Kcal
- Protein: 25g
- Carbohydrates: 30g
- Fat: 12g

Add Protein to Your Smoothie

3 TBSP WHOLE CHIA SEEDS 6 - 9 G PRO	3 TBSP SHELLED HEMP SEEDS 10 G PRO	3 TBSP HULLED SESAME SEEDS 7 G PRO	3 TBSP WHOLE FLAXSEEDS 6 - 8 G PRO
1 OZ RAW PISTACHIOS 6 G PRO	1/2 CUP UNCOOKED OATS 7 G PRO	1 CUP FLAX MILK 5 G PRO	1 OZ RAW ALMONDS 6 G PRO
1 WHOLE AVOCADO 3 G PRO	1 OZ CASHEWS 5 G PRO	1 OZ WALNUTS 4.5 G PRO	1 TBSP PEANUT BUTTER 4 G PRO
1 CUP BAKED SWEET POTATO 5 G PRO	1 CUP FROZEN TURNIP GREENS 6 G PRO	1 CUP FROZEN SPINACH 6 G PRO	1 CUP FROZEN CHERRIES 3 G PRO
1 CUP RAW BLACKBERRIES 2 G PRO	1 CUP RAW MULBERRIES 2 G PRO	2 LARGE KIWIFRUIT 2 G PRO	1 MEDIUM BANANA 1.5 G PRO

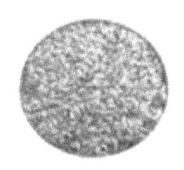

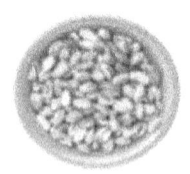

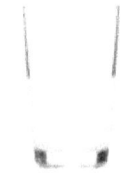

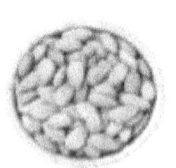

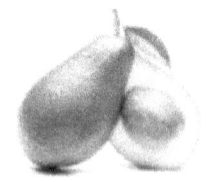

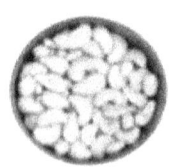

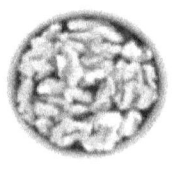

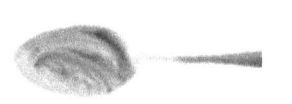

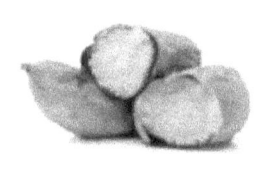

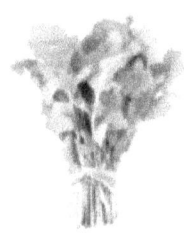

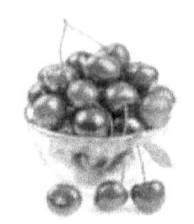

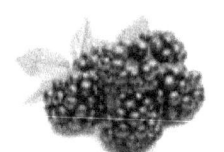

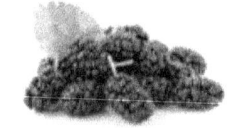

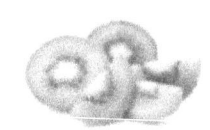

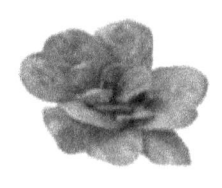

CPSIA information can be obtained
at www.ICGtesting.com
Printed in the USA
BVHW061443220621
610213BV00002B/408

9 781803 077116